PREGNANCY
DAY BY DAY

❖

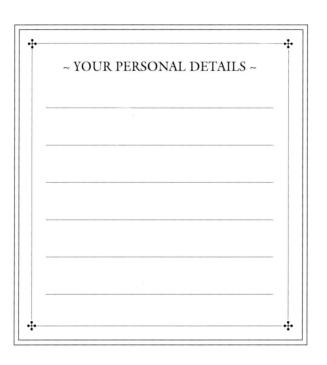

~ YOUR PERSONAL DETAILS ~

SHEILA KITZINGER
& VICKY BAILEY

PREGNANCY DAY BY DAY

❖

*The expectant mother's diary, record book,
and guide*

Photography by Nancy Durrell McKenna and Lennart Nilsson

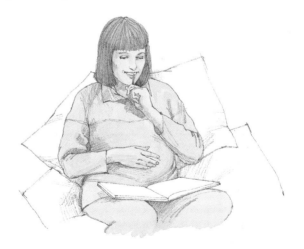

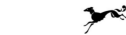

Alfred A. Knopf • New York • 2002

This is a Borzoi Book published by Alfred A. Knopf

Copyright © 1990 Dorling Kindersley Limited, London
Text copyright © 1990 Sheila Kitzinger & Vicky Bailey

www.sheilakitzinger.com

www.aaknopf.com
Knopf, Borzoi Books, and the colophon are registered trademarks of Random House, Inc.

Originaly published in Great Britain
by Dorling Kindersley Limited, London

Library of Congress Cataloging-in-Publication Data
Kitzinger, Sheila.
  Pregnancy day by day: a unique pregnancy diary, personal planner,
  and information-packed guide / Sheila Kitzinger & Vicky Bailey.
      p.   cm.
    Includes bibliographical references.
    ISBN 0-375-70945-2 pbk
    1. Pregnancy--Popular works. I. Bailey, Vicky. II. Title.
  RG525.K524   1990
  618.2'4--dc20   90-4508
                                                                     CIP
  LC: 90-053165

Consultant *Gerrianne Griffin Bodd, R N, BSN, CCE*

Page make-up by The Cooling Brown Partnership, Hersham, Surrey
Text film output by Manuscript Typesetting, Trowbridge, Wiltshire

Printed and bound in Singapore
by Star Standard Industries (PTE) Ltd.
Reproduction by Colourscan, Singapore

Published November 1, 1990
First Paperback Edition, February 2001
Second Printing, December 2002

CONTENTS

Introducing this Book ~ 6
You're Pregnant! ~ 8

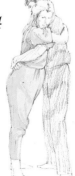
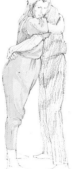
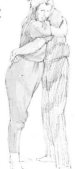

INTRODUCING THIS BOOK

LONG AFTER A BABY IS BORN, mothers often wish they could remember details of what happened and exactly how they felt during pregnancy and birth. They may want to share it with their child and be able to say, "This happened before you were born" or "The day you were born . . .". So this is a book not just to read. In these pages you can tell your own story of pregnancy and birth, record information you want to remember, and find out what you need to know at different stages of pregnancy. This book can help you write about a very important experience, and make your own unique and personal record of a special time in your life.

~ WHY WE WROTE THE BOOK ~

We both believe that birth is an important event for a woman, and that it should never be treated as just a medical matter. You have a right to full and accurate information to know the benefits and risks of things that are done to you and your baby. You can be an active birth-giver, not merely a passive patient. We know that birth can be an intensely exciting and deeply satisfying experience, and would like to help make it like that for you.

Week 17   MONTH / DAY / YEAR

S
M
T
W
T
F
S

Week 18   MONTH / DAY / YEAR

S
M
T
W
T
F
S

Notepads contain questions to stimulate thought and discussion.

DAY BY DAY DIARY *Here you can note dates and times of prenatal visits and other information.*

Body Facts panels detail changes in your body at each stage.

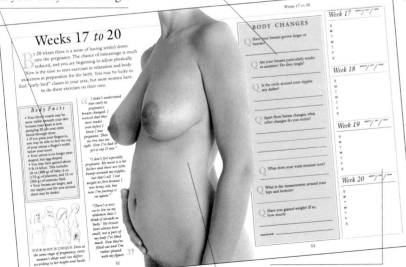

YOUR BODY *Two pages featuring a mother-to-be introduce each one of the book's nine sections.*

A day by day diary lets you record special dates.

Photographs of pregnant women help you discover your own body.

YOUR BABY *The two pages following* YOUR BODY *chart the baby from conception to birth.*

~ HOW THE BOOK WORKS ~

The book has nine sections, one for each stage of pregnancy, starting when you first realized you were pregnant and continuing through to the birth and your first meeting with your baby. YOUR BODY, at the beginning of each section, describes the changes you can expect in your body, with a day by day diary for noting appointments and special dates. Following this, YOUR BABY tells you how the baby is developing inside you. SPECIAL SUBJECTS in each section give you practical advice and information, and suggest topics for thought and discussion, while Notepads contain careful questions and provide space for you to write about your own experiences, describe your thoughts and feelings, and record decisions you have made about you and your baby.

~ ABOUT THE PHOTOGRAPHS ~

You may be anxious that the changes in your body are not normal. So the YOUR BODY pages show a specially commissioned photograph of a different woman at each stage of pregnancy. We hope these will help you to know and understand your own body.

NOTEPADS *Your thoughts, feelings, and decisions, written in response to the questions in these panels, will create a lasting record of your own personal experience of pregnancy and birth.*

THINKING ABOUT

Q How do you feel about breastfeeding?

_____

_____

_____

_____

_____

_____

Q Who can you contact for help with breas

Did You Know

• The tasty morsels in the amniotic fluid include glucose and fructose, salt, protein, urea, citric acid, lactic acid, fatty acids, and amino acids.

DID YOU KNOW
Fascinating facts reveal new insights into what the fetus can do, see, hear, and feel.

Did You Know panels tell you all about the baby.

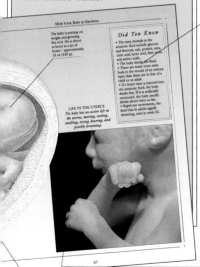

Amazing photographs of the fetus provide vivid detail.

Full-color drawings illustrate the developing baby at each stage.

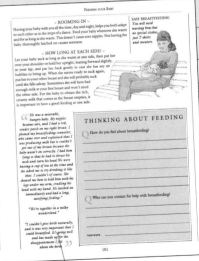

SPECIAL SUBJECTS *Advice and information are combined with complementary illustrations.*

Comments by other women add a unique dimension.

Features contain specific information.

You're Pregnant!

YOU MAY BE OVERJOYED to discover that you are pregnant. It seems incredible that life is growing inside you, and you feel like the first woman ever to be having a baby! Perhaps you conceived accidentally, or have been trying for ages. You may be delighted to find that your body is in working order, yet have doubts about whether you are ready to be a mother, or wonder how the baby will affect your relationship with your partner. Honestly accepting these mixed emotions is the best way to start out on this great adventure.

~ WHEN IS THE BABY DUE? ~

Pregnancy lasts 38 weeks, but medically the date on which the baby will be born is calculated as 40 weeks from the first day of your last period, two weeks before you *probably* ovulated. Since no one knows when you actually ovulated, and even you may not remember exactly when you made love, this date is only an estimate. The baby may be born two weeks before or after the expected date, and still be on time.

"I wanted the baby with Richard because, although I had a family already, he'd never had children. He's pleased as punch, and the other kids are delighted. I seem to have made a lot of people I love happy just by getting pregnant."

"I rushed out and bought books about childbirth. I bought a fuzzy duck, too. Part of me said: That's silly. What's a new baby going to do with a fuzzy duck, anyway?"

"I'd like to be a full-time mother if I can but I don't know how we're going to manage without my income. This is the most wonderful thing that has ever happened to me, and we'll find a way."

"My sister's a Down child, and I'm down-playing the whole idea of being pregnant until after I've had my amniocentesis. I don't want to tell other people yet, until I'm sure I'm going ahead."

A BABY! *Finding out you're pregnant may bring a flood of mixed emotions for you and your partner.*

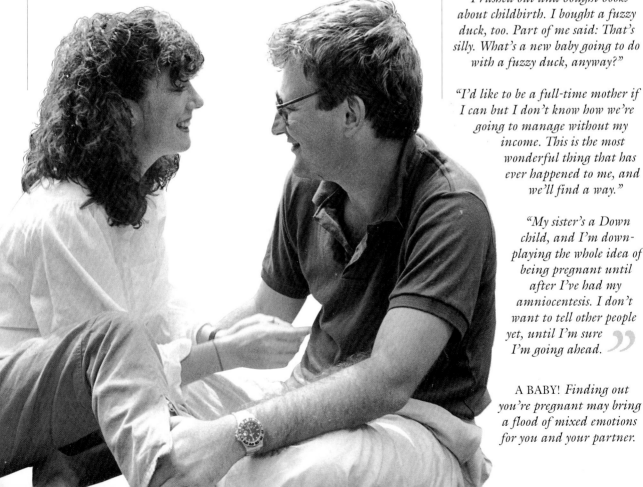

TELLING PEOPLE

Q How did you feel when you realized that you were pregnant?

_____
_____
_____
_____
_____

Q Who did you tell first about your pregnancy?

_____
_____
_____

Q When you gave the news that you were pregnant, what did you say?

_____
_____
_____

Q How did the person you told first react?

_____

Q Who was the second person you told about your pregnancy?

_____
_____
_____

Q How did the second person you told react?

_____
_____
_____

Q Has it been difficult to tell anyone that you're pregnant? If so, who and why?

_____
_____
_____
_____

TODAY'S DATE _____

Weeks 1 *to* 8

IT MAY SEEM AMAZING that you are walking around with a miracle unfolding inside you and no one is aware of it. You feel you must look different. But you don't. In the early weeks you may feel tired, as the way your body works adapts to the demands of pregnancy. You need extra rest, but because most people don't know you are pregnant it can be difficult to organize. See if you can get to bed early, and ask your partner to bring you breakfast in bed if possible. You may be able to enjoy lazy weekends together. During these first weeks you may have early morning or evening nausea, with or without vomiting. Or you may have a metallic taste in your mouth that sometimes lasts right through the day. These conditions can be caused by tiredness, and more rest will reduce the symptoms as well as prevent you from getting exhausted. There are other suggestions below that may help you to reduce nausea in these early weeks.

BODY AWARENESS
The changing shape and size of your body may be a source of fascination, as you contemplate the baby developing deep within you. Or you may worry about becoming "fat" and wonder if your partner will still find you attractive. Thinking positively, taking pride in your new rounded form, will help you to relax and feel more confident.

"I've started seeing pregnant women everywhere! They seem to be all around, and I wonder: Will I ever look like that? Will I ever really be that big?"

"I'm feeling run-down, but I realize that my body has to make an enormous adjustment, so I'm taking it easy for a few weeks.

Coping with Morning Sickness

• Have some dry toast *before* you lift your head from the pillow in the morning. This will boost your blood sugar level. Nausea occurs most commonly early in the morning when the level is low.
• Have a light snack before you go to bed.
• Eat small, frequent meals, high in carbohydrate. Something as simple as a banana will help to sustain your blood sugar level.
• Cut out fats and reduce the amount of whole milk, hard cheeses, and eggs in your diet.
• Eat graham crackers between meals so that your stomach is never empty.
• Suck peeled root ginger.
• For a day or so, eat only one food that you know you can keep down. Then add another, and so on.

• Avoid strong odors, hot stuffy rooms, and smoky atmospheres.
• Set aside a particular time each day to put your feet up.
• Ask your partner to share everyday household tasks.
• If you go out to work, try to negotiate flexible working hours with your employer.
• Discuss possible effects of anti-nausea medication on your baby with your doctor.

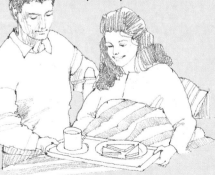

10

CHANGES IN YOUR BODY

Q What differences have you noticed in yourself since you found out that you were pregnant?

_____

_____

_____

_____

_____

_____

_____

_____

_____

_____

_____

_____

_____

_____

_____

_____

_____

TODAY'S DATE _____

Week 1   MONTH / DAY / YEAR

S
M
T
W
T
F
S

Week 2   MONTH / DAY / YEAR

S
M
T
W
T
F
S

Week 3   MONTH / DAY / YEAR

S
M
T
W
T
F
S

Week 4   MONTH / DAY / YEAR

S
M
T
W
T
F
S

Week 5   MONTH / DAY / YEAR

S
M
T
W
T
F
S

Week 6   MONTH / DAY / YEAR

S
M
T
W
T
F
S

Week 7   MONTH / DAY / YEAR

S
M
T
W
T
F
S

Week 8   MONTH / DAY / YEAR

S
M
T
W
T
F
S

THE FIRST WEEKS

Y OUR EGG, OR OVUM, is ready to be fertilized by sperm for only 12 to 24 hours. Egg and sperm meet in one of the two fallopian tubes. The sperm burrows its head into the ovum, its tail drops off, and the ovum absorbs it. In two to three hours the ovum divides into two cells. In three days it splits into 32 cells, and by the fifth day into 90 cells. The cell cluster bounces down the tube towards your uterus, squeezed in the right direction by the tube, and helped by long cells which sweep it along like a field of wheat blowing in the wind.

~ HOW THE EMBRYO DEVELOPS ~

About a week after sperm and ovum have fused, the cell cluster – still only just visible to the naked eye – implants in the lining of your uterus. One layer of cells absorbs some of the lining, grows into it, and gets a firm hold. Another layer becomes a protective bag of waters which grows and surrounds the embryo. In the middle of the cell cluster is the part that will later be the baby, and a yolk sac that produces red blood cells and later becomes part of the baby's gut.

BOY OR GIRL?

M ost women discover the sex of their baby at birth, although it can be established by amniocentesis (see page 34), CVS (see page 35), or ultrasound (see page 46). The father's sperm determines if it is a boy or a girl.

The ovum always carries two X chromosomes, but the sperm carries either an X or a Y chromosome. If a Y sperm fertilized your ovum you will have a boy, and if it was an X sperm, you will have a girl.

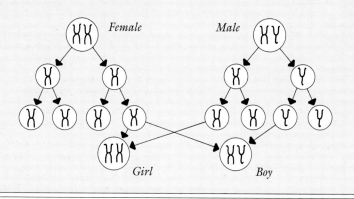

Female   Male

Girl   Boy

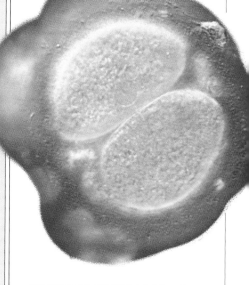

IN THE BEGINNING *The ripe egg* (top left), *released from an ovary, divides into two cells* (above) *a few hours after fertilization.*

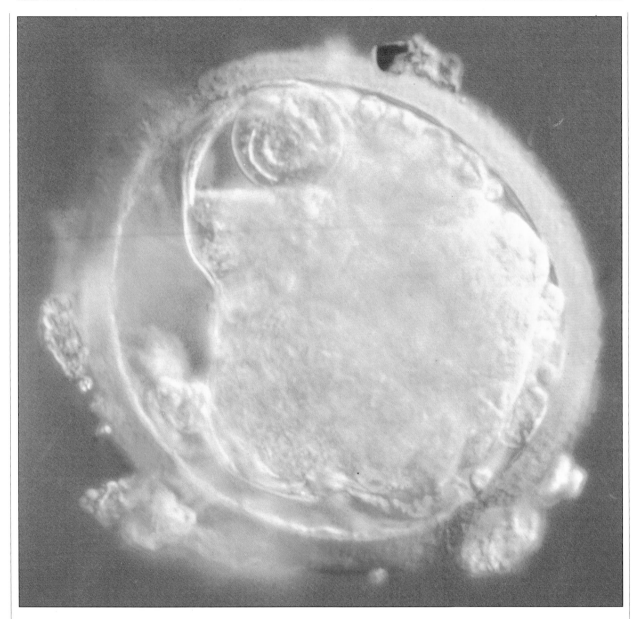

DATING YOUR PREGNANCY

The embryonic disc has turned into an embryo by what is accepted as the eighth week of pregnancy. In fact, it is six weeks after conception. Although you have been pregnant only six weeks, it is conventional to call it eight weeks because pregnancy is dated from the first day of your last period, not from when you actually started the baby.

Did You Know

• The embryo is connected to the placenta (*see* page 41) by a thin stalk. As the embryo grows it is formed like a soap bubble when you blow it from a pipe. It swells from inside and becomes longer.

• The embryo has 3 layers of tissues, which develop separately.

• The outer layer grows into the baby's skin and nerves.

• The middle layer grows into cartilage, bones, connective tissues, muscles, the circulatory system, kidneys, and sex organs.

• The inner layer grows into the organs of breathing and digestion.

INFORMED DECISIONS

IT MAKES SENSE to think as early as possible about the kind of care you want during pregnancy and how you would like the birth of your baby to be. To come to these decisions, you will need a great deal of information – from your doctor and midwife, the hospital, and your local childbirth group. It is useful to talk to friends and other women who have had babies, too, so ask them about their experiences of pregnancy and birth. To help you think through the things that are important to you, discuss them with your partner or someone else close to you, and read some of the books listed on page 126. When you have found out everything you need to know, write your answers to the questions on pages 16–17 so that you have a personal record.

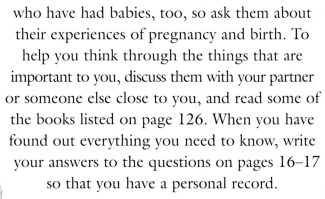

Getting information . . .

"I started off thinking: They know best. But I came to realize that I know more about my body and myself – what I'm capable of – than they do. My obstetrician said: 'This is a very precious baby, and because of your age [I'm 40] we'll have you in for a Cesarean section.' I asked him, 'Is there any other reason why you think I need surgery?' 'No indications,' he said, 'but you can't expect your body to work as well as a younger woman's.' I said, 'Thank you, but no. I appreciate your caring, but I'm fit – in fact, I feel healthier than before I was pregnant; I swim every day – and I want to have this baby as naturally as possible.' "

"I know that my body will work better if I have a home birth. I'll be able to relax more. I was sexually abused as a child. I know that's happened to many women, but I don't want to be labeled as a victim by my doctor, so, although he's very nice, I'm not comfortable talking to him about that. Although I realize there are risk factors in my case, I've opted for home birth for very important personal reasons. "

~ YOUR CAREGIVERS ~

Although the kind of care available to you depends partly on where you live, the main choice you have is between a specialist who is part of a health insurance plan or in private practice; community care with a general practitioner and a midwife; and a midwife or team of midwives. Your own doctor may offer care during pregnancy and after birth, but not at the actual birth. You may feel that you do not want this particular doctor to care for you at this time, and want to be transferred to one who practices obstetrics. You may prefer to be cared for by a woman. But remember that there are far more men than women obstetricians.

If you want midwife care, find out what medical back-up facilities are available if the pregnancy or birth is complicated. Trained midwives are experts in normal childbirth and can also cope with a wide range of abnormal situations and emergencies with medical back-up.

~ GAINING CONFIDENCE ~

You may feel more confident if you hand over decisions about your care entirely to your caregivers. Or you may not want to hand over such important decisions to other people, and wish to be consulted about everything that is done to you, and share in the decision-making. Think about what feels right for you.

" I told the doctor I wanted to be sure I could have an epidural. He said, 'If you come in to be induced. Otherwise we can't guarantee one because the anesthetist is here only on Tuesdays, Thursdays, and Fridays.' That seemed like the wrong reason for having an induction, so I switched to another hospital."

"It's fine to talk about choices, but this is my first baby and I found it difficult to get the information I needed to make them. When I asked questions, the doctor said, 'Don't worry'. It was only when I started going to classes that I could discuss subjects like episiotomy."

~ INTERVENTIONS ~

Interventions in birth include artificial rupture of the membranes or a synthetic hormone drip either to start or to speed up labor; an intravenous drip to feed glucose into the bloodstream; and forceps, vacuum extraction, and episiotomy (being cut) to help get the baby out. Even commanded pushing to hasten the second stage imposes management techniques on a woman's spontaneous rhythms. In some hospitals, many of these interventions are used routinely.

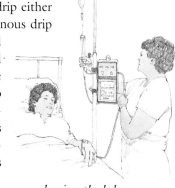

. . . having the labor . . .

~ CHOOSING A BIRTH PARTNER ~

Your birth partner is the person you choose as your main support, who should understand your wishes and share with you all the preparation for labor. It may be the father of your baby, a woman friend, or a relative. The important thing is that it is your choice, and that you do not feel bound to have someone simply because they are close to you.

. . . and birth partner you want . . .

~ HANDLING PAIN ~

Pain during labor and birth is very different from the pain you feel when you break a leg or have toothache. If you think of it as "pain with a purpose", you can find ways to work with it. In childbirth classes you will learn how to control pain yourself using relaxation and breathing, to open your pelvis wide and get into comfortable positions, and to visualize the power of your uterus sweeping through your body as the baby is pressed lower. Or you may decide to use drugs. But remember that all drugs have potential harmful side effects, for you and the baby.

~ THE BIRTH PLACE ~

The place where you have your baby is closely linked to your choice of caregivers. Doctors practice mostly in hospitals. Midwives practice both at home and in the hospital. Ask to see the birth place and any equipment that may be used before you come to your final decision.

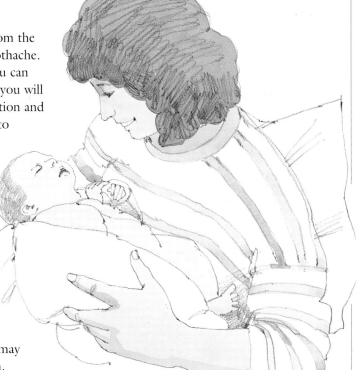

. . . at last you hold your baby in your arms.

YOUR CHOICES

Q During pregnancy and birth, would you prefer to be consulted about everything that is done to you, and to share in the decision-making? If so, why?

_____

_____

_____

_____

_____

_____

IMPORTANT DECISIONS *Take time to think through what your priorities are.*

Q Who would you like to care for you during pregnancy?

_____

_____

_____

Q Would you prefer to leave decisions about your care entirely to the professionals? If so, why?

_____

_____

_____

_____

_____

Q Who would you like to care for you at your baby's birth?

_____

_____

_____

Q If you want to take responsibility for your own body and for your baby, who can help you find out what you need to know?

_____

_____

_____

Q What are your feelings about interventions in childbirth?

_____

_____

_____

Q Would you like a support person (birth partner) with you at your baby's birth?

_____

_____

_____

Q If you do want a support person, who would you like this to be?

_____

_____

_____

Q Do you want to learn ways of handling and easing pain yourself?

_____

_____

_____

Q Would you prefer to take advantage of drugs to relieve pain?

_____

_____

Q If you have a choice, in what kind of setting would you like your baby to be born?

_____

_____

Q Are there other things that are important to you about your pregnancy and the birth?

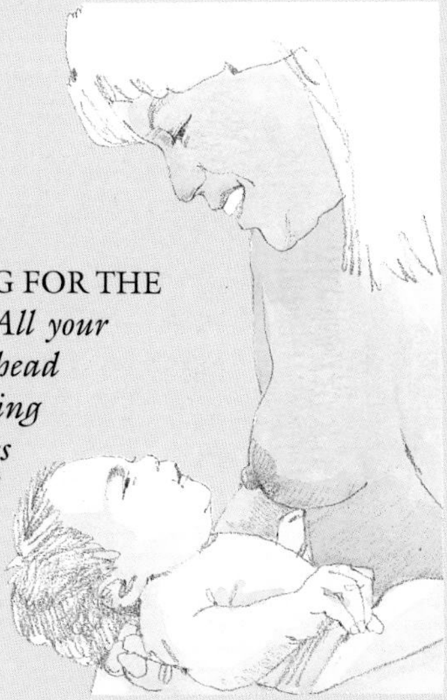

_____

_____

_____

_____

PLANNING FOR THE FUTURE *All your thinking ahead and exploring alternatives will be well worth it.*

TODAY'S DATE _____

THE BIRTH PLACE

EPENDING ON WHERE YOU LIVE, you can have your baby in a large hospital, a small hospital, a birth center, or at home. However, because many small hospitals are being closed down and women are required to travel to large hospitals, you may not have as much choice as you would like.

~ EXPLORING CHOICES ~

A large hospital has all the equipment needed for monitoring and dealing with complicated labor and birth. There is a special-care nursery where babies who are pre-term or ill can be treated. You may be able to choose between staying in full time and having early discharge.

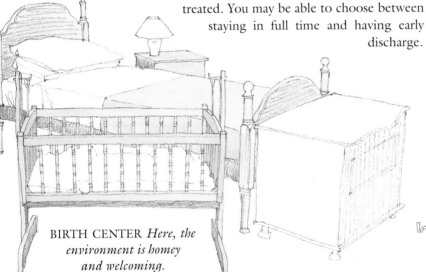

BIRTH CENTER *Here, the environment is homey and welcoming.*

> ### *Did You Know?*
>
> • It is as safe to give birth at home as in a hospital if your pregnancy is low-risk.
> • Some hospitals have birthing rooms with soft lighting, and, occasionally, double beds.
> • If you wish to have an epidural, you must find out which hospitals near your home provide this service.
> • A Birth Plan (*see* pages 80–81) enables doctors and midwives to help you have the kind of birth you want.

In a small hospital or birth center there is a more homey, relaxed atmosphere, and you are usually cared for by the same people who have provided your care during pregnancy. Some birth centers are adjacent to, or part of, a large hospital. Others are distant.

At home you are on your own ground, and the people who come to help you – already well-known to you – are there as your guests. Birth takes place within the family, and your other children can be present. If you decide on home birth, or choose early discharge from hospital, you will need good help after the baby is born.

~ MAKING A DECISION ~

Talk to other mothers about where they have given birth and what the experience was like for them. Get more information from local childbirth groups, midwives in your area, and your doctor. (*See also* pages 126–127 for useful books and organizations.) It is a good idea to explore all the options before you decide what is best for you and your baby.

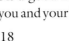

"I'd only feel safe in a hospital. I like the idea of a team of experts bringing their skills to the birth."

"Our birth center is very friendly – more like a comfortable small hotel than a hospital. There's very little intervention in birth and you don't get strung up to all those machines."

"I'm having a home birth because here I feel I can relax completely and trust my body to give birth in my own way and in my own time."

"I wanted to shop around before I chose. It meant joining a new mothers' network so that I could ask questions of women who had given birth in different places and with different doctors and midwives. Now I feel much better informed."

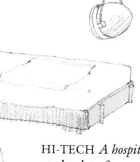

HI-TECH *A hospital has the technology for emergencies.*

YOUR BABY'S BIRTH PLACE

Q What birth place have you chosen and why?

_____

_____

_____

_____

_____

_____

Q If you are having a hospital birth, would you prefer to stay in full time or to have early discharge?

_____

_____

_____

_____

_____

_____

Q If you are having early discharge or home birth, who will help you after the baby is born?

_____

_____

_____

_____

TODAY'S DATE _____

PRENATAL CARE

THE TERM PRENATAL CARE usually means your care in pregnancy by doctors and midwives whom you see regularly. You will have regular checks on your health by means of routine tests (*see* pages 22–23) with special tests if you need them (*see* pages 34–35). Of course, professional help can only serve as a back-up to self-help and the support you get from family and friends.

There was a lot of hanging around at the clinic. The hospital leaflet said you could talk to other women and watch a video about birth. But we were all too anxious about missing our turn when they called out our names – so we just sat and waited.

~ YOUR CAREGIVERS ~

Your first visit to your doctor is exciting because you may already know you are pregnant, or even discover it then. Your doctor discusses with you where you would like to have your baby, and who will look after you.

Most women have hospital care. One option may be to have your baby in a hospital under the supervision of an obstetrician, but get most of your care from a midwife at the hospital or doctor's office. Some doctors or midwives provide all your care and deliver you at a birth center backed up by a hospital and obstetrician, whom you may see once or twice during your pregnancy. In many group insurance plans, women visit a clinic and see any number of doctors during their pregnancies. Find out what other choices you have.

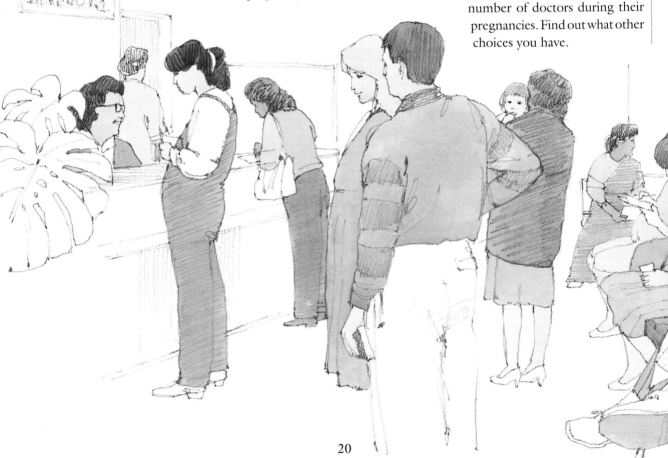

He seemed to be looking for everything and anything that could possibly go wrong. I went in feeling healthy and normal and came out feeling high-risk. Then I called my local childbirth group and talked to a woman who says he's always like that."

"Going to the doctor made me feel special. I was so busy at work that those spaces just for me and the baby were precious."

"I enjoyed it. A midwife sat down with you and explained things and found out what you wanted. She was so friendly. You wouldn't have thought anyone was having a baby except me!"

POINT OF CONTACT *At a prenatal clinic you may be able to talk to other women and make new friends.*

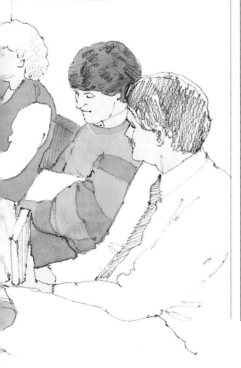

~ VISITING THE DOCTOR ~

When you know you are pregnant you can begin to make arrangements for prenatal care. Most women have their first check between 12 and 16 weeks. After this you usually see your doctor or midwife every four weeks until 28 weeks, every two weeks between 28 and 36 weeks, and weekly from 36 weeks until the birth.

At your first visit you are asked questions about yourself, your family, your medical background, and any previous pregnancies. You are examined and some routine tests are done. The results are recorded (*see* page 24) in your notes, which are put in a folder. Visiting the doctor gives you regular opportunities to discuss your care (and any problems) with your caregivers.

AT THE DOCTOR'S OFFICE

Q Was your first visit for prenatal care what you expected?

_____

_____

Q What were your feelings about your first prenatal visit?

_____

_____

_____

Q Did you have an opportunity to discuss all the things you wanted to?

_____

Q What questions do you want to ask on your next visit?

_____

_____

_____

_____

TODAY'S DATE _____

ROUTINE TESTS

ROUTINE TESTS ARE PERFORMED REGULARLY throughout your pregnancy and are a way of monitoring that you and your baby are keeping healthy. They can take place at the medical facility or in your home. If any problems occur, your doctor and midwife will keep a closer eye on you, and carry out special tests (*see* pages 34–35) if you need them.

~ TAKING BLOOD PRESSURE AND TESTING URINE ~

Your blood pressure is taken every time you see your doctor or midwife because a minority of women have raised or high blood pressure, which can develop into pre-eclampsia (*see* page 92). Your blood pressure may rise simply because you are tense or anxious – perhaps as a result of a long wait in a crowded waiting room. If this is the case ask your doctor or midwife to check it at home where you are more relaxed.

Urine tests are important because they may reveal signs of infection. Protein in the urine may be a sign of pre-eclampsia (*see* page 92) or infection. Sugar found in repeated urine tests may be a sign of diabetes. The occasional trace of sugar may simply be the result of eating a sweet food, like a banana.

TIME FACTOR
Blood pressure is lowest early in the day.

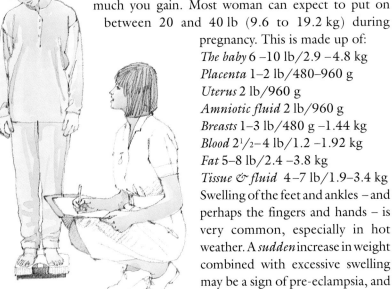

> *I was determined to ask questions about everything, and not just have things happen to me without understanding why. The nurse said, 'It's wonderful having someone really interested', and she explained it all fully.*

"I expected to be able to have a real conversation about my pregnancy, but each time they rush me through with reassuring noises. I've written a letter to the doctor to say I'd appreciate the opportunity to have a discussion next time and find out more about what's happening."

LOSING WEIGHT *Avoid reducing diets in pregnancy.*

~ GAINING WEIGHT ~

Weight gain is an issue that always causes discussion. It seems that no one knows whether or not it is really important how much you gain. Most woman can expect to put on between 20 and 40 lb (9.6 to 19.2 kg) during pregnancy. This is made up of:

The baby 6 –10 lb/2.9 –4.8 kg
Placenta 1–2 lb/480–960 g
Uterus 2 lb/960 g
Amniotic fluid 2 lb/960 g
Breasts 1–3 lb/480 g –1.44 kg
Blood $2\frac{1}{2}$–4 lb/1.2 –1.92 kg
Fat 5–8 lb/2.4 –3.8 kg
Tissue & fluid 4–7 lb/1.9–3.4 kg
Swelling of the feet and ankles – and perhaps the fingers and hands – is very common, especially in hot weather. A *sudden* increase in weight combined with excessive swelling may be a sign of pre-eclampsia, and will need attention.

GIVING BLOOD
A blood test only takes a minute.

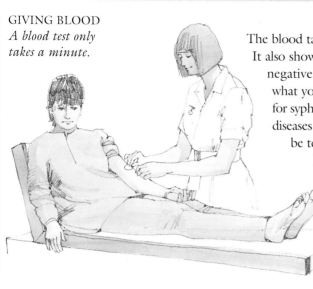

~ TESTING BLOOD ~

The blood taken at your first prenatal visit reveals your blood group. It also shows whether you are Rhesus positive (like most people) or negative, if you are immune to rubella (German measles), and what your hemoglobin (iron count) is. Your blood is also tested for syphilis and hepatitis virus, a liver disease. Although rare, these diseases may be transmitted to the baby. In some states you may be tested for HIV antibodies (AIDS).

If you are Rhesus negative and the baby's father is Rhesus positive, blood tests at later visits in pregnancy will show if you have made antibodies (see page 51). All women have their hemoglobin monitored because its level tends to fall naturally in pregnancy. To help your hemoglobin level, eat more iron-rich foods such as green leafy vegetables, apricots, firmly cooked egg yolk, and whole grains.

WHAT IS PALPATION?

Throughout your pregnancy your midwife and doctor will palpate your abdomen regularly, using touch to see how your uterus and baby are growing. A large uterus may be the first sign that you are expecting twins.

After 20 weeks they feel for your baby's head, bottom, limbs, and back, to try to work out which way the baby is lying and whether its size is right for this stage of pregnancy. The baby changes position many times, but after 34 weeks tends to stay either head- or bottom-down (see pages 98–99).

Your caregivers watch the way the baby tumbles around the uterus, and listen to its heartbeat. Vigorous movements and a strong heart are signs of its wellbeing. In the last weeks your caregivers feel how deeply your baby's head or bottom has settled into your pelvis.

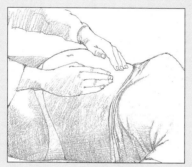
Your caregiver feels for the top of your uterus, to check that it is the right size.

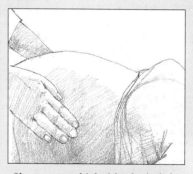
She sees on which side the baby's back is lying. You might feel the baby kicking on the opposite side.

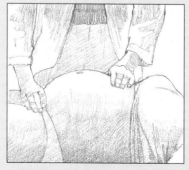
She checks the baby's size, and whether the baby is lying head- or bottom-down.

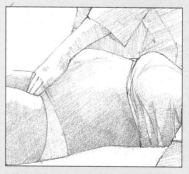
She feels to see if any part of the baby's head or bottom has entered your pelvis.

DECODING YOUR RECORDS

EACH TIME YOU GO FOR A PRENATAL VISIT, information about your pregnancy is recorded in a folder, which is kept in the doctor's office. If you are having care from the hospital and a midwife, the results of routine tests are sent to your midwife at your request. You have the right to read these records and have them photocopied for your own information. However, many of the terms may not make much sense, as they are abbreviated. The table below contains those that are most commonly used.

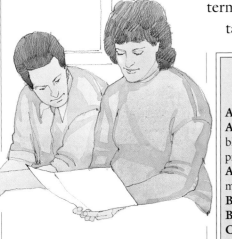

KEEPING AN EYE ON PROGRESS *You can see for yourself how your pregnancy is going by reading through your records.*

It's really good at my hospital clinic. They have a wall chart that tells you what everything means. It gives you something to look at while you're waiting to be seen.

"Why can't they use plain words instead of jargon, and explain what they mean?"

ABBREVIATIONS AND TERMS

AF   Artificial feeding.
APH   Antepartum hemorrhage: bleeding after 28 weeks of pregnancy.
ARM   Artificial rupture of membranes.
BP   Blood pressure.
Br   Breech: bottom-first.
Ceph   Cephalic: head-first.
CRL   Crown to rump length: length of the fetus from the top of its head to its bottom.
CS   Cesarean section.
Cx   Cervix.
EDC/EDD   Expected date of confinement/Expected date of delivery.
Eng   Engaged: where the head or the bottom is deep in the pelvis.
FH   Fetal heart.
FHR   Fetal heart rate.
FHHR   Fetal heart heard and regular.
Hb   Hemoglobin: contained in the blood. Women with low levels may need iron supplements.
Hct   Hematocrit of the blood. This is another way of measuring iron levels.
HIV$^{(+)(-)}$ The presence or absence in the blood of antibodies to the AIDS virus.
IOL   Induction of labor.

LSCS   Lower segment Cesarean section.
Misc   Miscarriage.
MSU   Mid-stream specimen of urine.
Multip   Woman who has already had a baby.
NAD   Nothing abnormal detected.
NICU   Neonatal intensive care unit.
P + M   Placenta and membranes.
PET   Pre-eclamptic toxemia.
PNH   Prenatal hemorrhage: bleeding after 28 weeks of pregnancy.
PP   Presenting part: the part of the baby over the cervix.
PPH   Postpartum hemorrhage: excessive bleeding at any time during the puerperium.
Primip   Woman expecting her first baby.
Puerperium   A period of six weeks after the birth of the baby.
Rh+/Rh–   The presence or absence in the blood of the Rhesus factor.
SA   Spontaneous abortion: a miscarriage
SB   Stillbirth.
SCBU   Special care baby unit.
SROM   Spontaneous rupture of membranes.
TOP   Termination of pregnancy.
USS   Ultrasound scan.
Vx   Vertex: head-down.

LOSING A BABY

EVERYWHERE IN THE WORLD birth represents hope and thanksgiving. It is part of the onward flow of life: to be pregnant is to be ripe; to give birth is to be fruitful. When pregnancy fails through miscarriage, or with the death of a baby at birth, it is as if the natural order of things has come to a stop.

~ WHY DOES MISCARRIAGE HAPPEN? ~

Most miscarriages occur in the first 12 weeks of pregnancy. Usually no one knows the reason, although probably something was wrong with the chromosomes – the parts of the cell carrying the genes that determine what the baby will be like. Sometimes the cell cluster can't get enough nourishment from the lining of the uterus because a woman's hormone balance is not quite right, and so is unable to develop.

~ UNDERSTANDING YOUR FEELINGS ~

Miscarriage can be a shattering experience, and not only because it means the death of a baby. When you lose a baby you feel different from other women. If it was your first pregnancy, it may make you question whether you will ever manage to become a mother. You may not be able to bear seeing pregnant women or babies. You grieve for the baby that you have lost, and wonder what it would have been like, and you grieve for the loss of yourself as a mother. Knowing that you may have these feelings prepares you to face and accept them, and can give you strength.

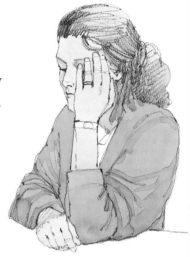

FEELING ALONE *As a result of your loss you may feel separated from women who have children.*

Preparing for your Next Pregnancy

Here are some things that are worth considering before you plan your next pregnancy.
• A woman who smokes runs a much greater risk of miscarriage than a woman who doesn't. (She also risks having a premature baby or one that doesn't grow well inside the uterus.)
• Giving up smoking a few months before you plan to conceive will give your next pregnancy a better chance. Tips for how to give up are on page 33.
• Breaking the habit may also help to improve your general health.

• Think about nutrition: a balanced and varied diet helps your body to work efficiently.
• Have a look at the list of good foods on page 31.
• Foods rich in zinc may help your baby's development. Good sources include wheat bran, oatmeal, wholemeal flour, brewer's yeast, sesame seeds, egg yolk (well cooked), and some cheeses, such as Edam and Cheddar.

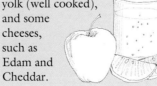

"*I can't trust my body any more. I've always been able to rely on it before, but now it's as if I'm handicapped. I think it'll take some time for me to get over that feeling, and only having a successful pregnancy will make me feel confident again.*"

"*Stephen wouldn't discuss our baby's death, and thought the sooner we could forget it the better. I needed to talk about her, to have photographs of her around, and that upset him. But now we're seeing a bereavement counselor and she's helped us to understand that we each need to grieve in our own way.*"

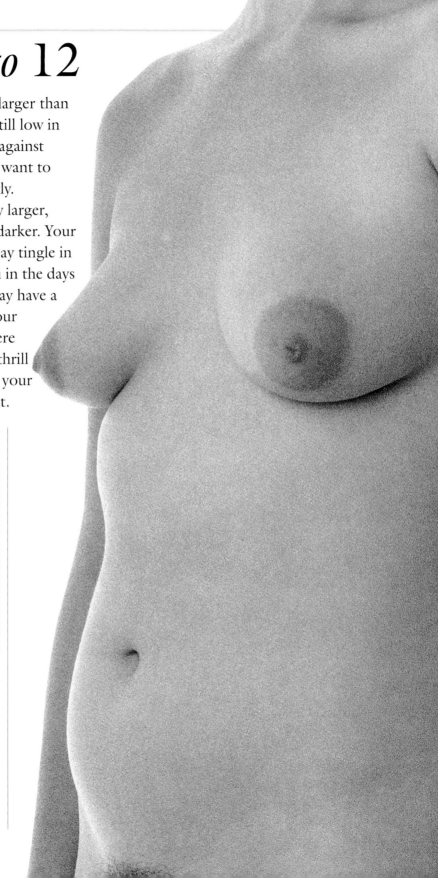

Weeks 9 *to* 12

Y OUR UTERUS is a little larger than a tennis ball now. It is still low in your pelvis and presses against your bladder so that you want to urinate more frequently.

Your nipples are probably larger, and the circles around them darker. Your breasts are fuller, and they may tingle in a way that was familiar to you in the days just before a period. You may have a sense of fullness low in your abdomen, too, as if you were about to start a period. The thrill of being pregnant may make your whole body feel vibrant.

Sex in Pregnancy

• Some women lose interest in sex because they are tired, or nauseated, or feel protective about the baby.
• A man may be anxious that he might hurt the baby.
• Sex is not just about intercourse. It is about your total relationship – the way you touch, look at, speak to, and care for each other.

I had a miscarriage last time, so I am taking life very calmly and not getting worked up about anything.

"I just flop into bed when I come home from the office, and stay there. Sex is out of the question. Pete gives me a terrific back-rub instead!"

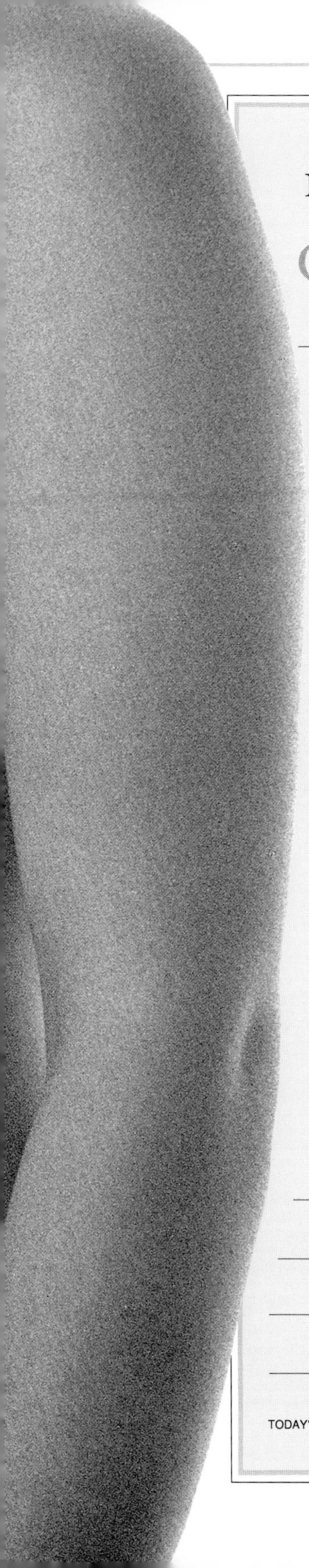

PHYSICAL AND EMOTIONAL CHANGES

Q Do you notice any changes in your breasts?

_____

Q Are you aware of any other physical changes?

_____

_____

Q Has pregnancy changed your relationship with your partner in any way?

_____

_____

_____

_____

_____

_____

Q Has being pregnant affected your feelings about sex?

_____

_____

_____

_____

TODAY'S DATE _____

Week 9 MONTH / DAY / YEAR

S
M
T
W
T
F
S

Week 10 MONTH / DAY / YEAR

S
M
T
W
T
F
S

Week 11 MONTH / DAY / YEAR

S
M
T
W
T
F
S

Week 12 MONTH / DAY / YEAR

S
M
T
W
T
F
S

HOW YOUR BABY IS GROWING

BY 12 WEEKS sexual differentiation has taken place and the embryo has developed the organs that will show that it is male or female. The kidneys have formed and the embryo starts to pass urine into the amniotic fluid in which it floats. The eyelids have developed and the eyes, which were previously lidless, are closed. Tooth buds are forming and the vocal cords are beginning to develop.

The baby begins to move, at first with twitches and trembles that start in the arms and legs and spread to the neck and trunk. Then it begins to bend and stretch its legs, to make stepping movements, to make a fist and open its hands, and to lift and lower its head. Yet it is still far too small for you to feel these movements.

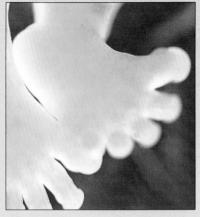

EXERCISING THE BODY
The baby develops its muscles through vigorous exercise in the uterus. It can move easily because it is floating in the amniotic fluid.

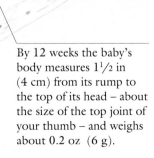

At 9 weeks the baby's hand measures $^1/4$ in (6 mm) – about the size of a pea.

By 12 weeks the baby's body measures $1^1/2$ in (4 cm) from its rump to the top of its head – about the size of the top joint of your thumb – and weighs about 0.2 oz (6 g).

Did You Know

• At this stage the baby is in the top part of your uterus only. The lower part above your cervix – the mouth of the uterus – gets very soft, so it is as if the baby were nestled on top of a large, soft cushion.
• The amniotic fluid in which the baby floats is enriched salt water. Nutrients in this fluid diffuse through the baby's skin, which is only a few cells thick, and are absorbed by the baby.

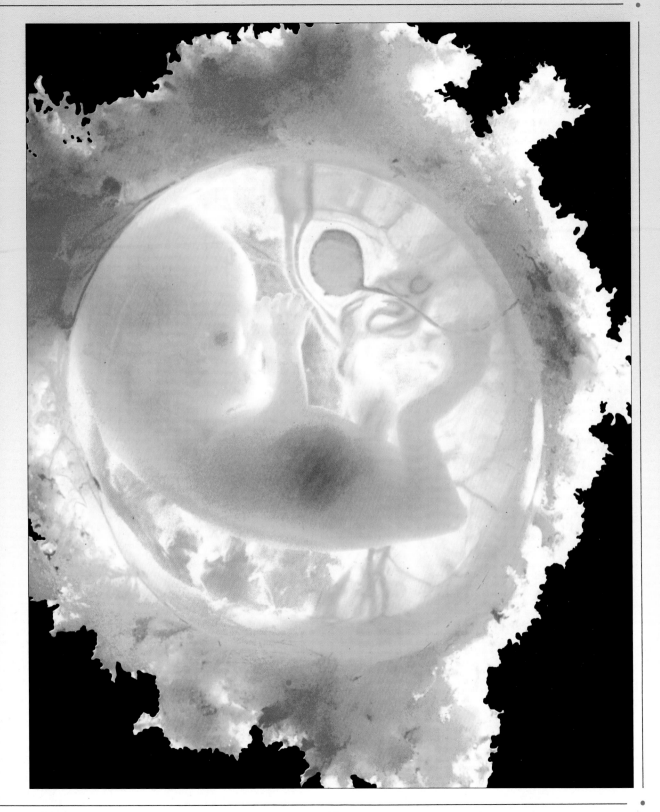

EATING WELL

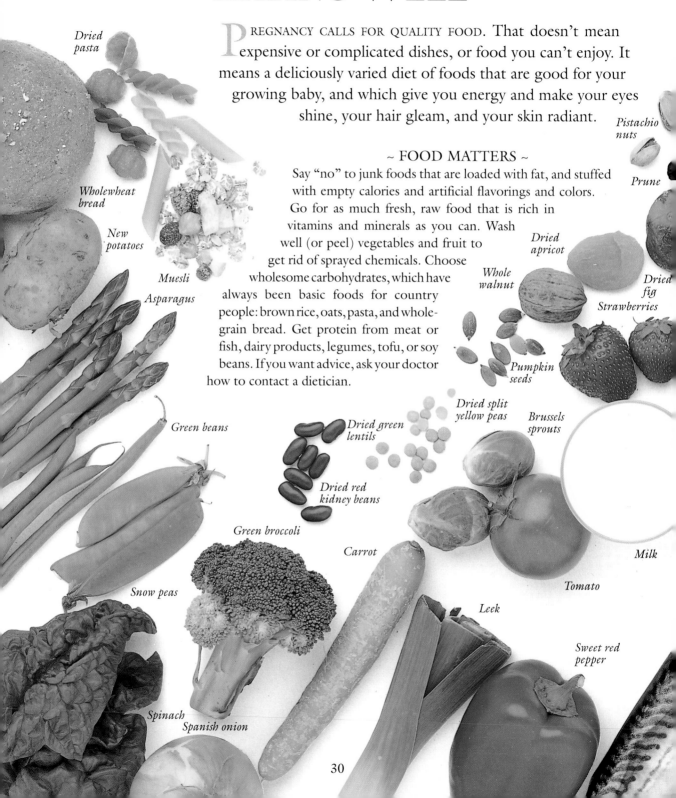

Pregnancy calls for quality food. That doesn't mean expensive or complicated dishes, or food you can't enjoy. It means a deliciously varied diet of foods that are good for your growing baby, and which give you energy and make your eyes shine, your hair gleam, and your skin radiant.

~ FOOD MATTERS ~

Say "no" to junk foods that are loaded with fat, and stuffed with empty calories and artificial flavorings and colors. Go for as much fresh, raw food that is rich in vitamins and minerals as you can. Wash well (or peel) vegetables and fruit to get rid of sprayed chemicals. Choose wholesome carbohydrates, which have always been basic foods for country people: brown rice, oats, pasta, and whole-grain bread. Get protein from meat or fish, dairy products, legumes, tofu, or soy beans. If you want advice, ask your doctor how to contact a dietician.

Dried pasta

Wholewheat bread

New potatoes

Muesli

Asparagus

Pistachio nuts

Prune

Dried apricot

Whole walnut

Dried fig

Strawberries

Pumpkin seeds

Green beans

Dried green lentils

Dried split yellow peas

Brussels sprouts

Dried red kidney beans

Green broccoli

Carrot

Milk

Snow peas

Tomato

Leek

Sweet red pepper

Spinach

Spanish onion

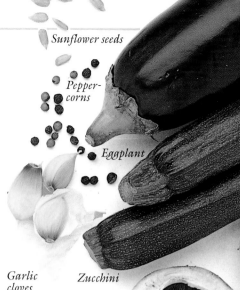

Sunflower seeds

Pepper-corns

Eggplant

~ MAKING CHANGES ~

To keep up your energy, it is better to have frequent snacks of quality foods such as nuts, raisins, or fresh fruit, than two solid meals a day. The hormone progesterone relaxes the bowel muscles in pregnancy, so some women become constipated. To avoid this, drink plenty of fluids, and eat prunes and high-fiber cereals. If you have indigestion, cut down on fatty foods, and eat slowly. Diluting wine with sparkling mineral water reduces alcohol intake. If you like coffee, drink only decaffeinated. Choose mineral water or fruit juice instead of synthetically flavored and colored drinks or sodas.

If your partner or friend will shop or cook for you, you can enjoy some especially relaxed meals that you have not had to prepare yourself.

Almond

Filberts

Plum

Red grapes

Lime

Green grapes

Apple

Garlic cloves

Zucchini

Mushrooms

CHOOSING GOOD FOODS

Here is a list of some good foods for pregnancy.
Check those you eat twice a week or more.

CARBOHYDRATES
Whole-grain bread □ Potatoes □
Brown rice □ Pasta □ Oats □

IRON-RICH FOODS
Green leafy vegetables □
Lentils □ Eggs □
Dried fruit □ Red meat □

VITAMIN-RICH FOODS
Citrus fruit □ Potatoes □
Tomatoes □ Berries □

PROTEIN
Milk □ Cheese □ Yogurt □
Lean meat □ Fish □ Tofu □
Nuts □ Legumes □

Q What did you eat and drink yesterday?

_____

_____

_____

_____

_____

TODAY'S DATE _____

Mackerel

Parsley

Cheddar cheese

NEW TASTES
A good diet is varied. Enjoy herbs, nuts, and spices, too.

NURTURING YOUR BABY

TODAY, CHILDBIRTH IS SAFER than it ever has been before, yet this does not mean that pregnant women worry any less that harm might come to their unborn babies. In fact, one kind of anxiety is more marked nowadays than it was in the past. We can hardly open our newspapers without reading about some new environmental hazard. It seems as if we cannot avoid entirely chemicals and bacteria in the food we eat, the water we drink, even the air we breathe, however careful we are as individuals. Thinking about these things can be alarming for a pregnant woman. Yet there are steps you can take for your own well-being, and to make your uterus as safe a place as possible for your baby.

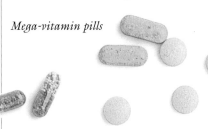

Mega-vitamin pills

Common cold treatments

~ EARLY DEVELOPMENT ~

During the first eight weeks of pregnancy, the main organs of the baby's body are being formed. If healthy development is affected then, miscarriage may result, or sometimes the heart, lungs, kidneys, brain, eyes, or palate of the mouth may be damaged. After this time there is much less risk, but *concentrated* poisons can still lead to premature birth, reduce growth, or harm the baby's later mental development and behavior. So, in order to protect the baby inside you, there are some things that you may decide to avoid while you are pregnant.

~ TAKING CONTROL ~

Ask your doctor if any prescribed medicines you may be taking are harmful to the baby. For many drugs, there is insufficient information to answer that question with any certainty. But if the answer is "yes," these medicines can usually be changed to others that are much more likely to be safe in pregnancy. If a drug is known to have damaging effects, but is the best one to treat you, discuss with your doctor the pros and cons of not having this treatment, compared with those of taking the drug. This isn't a matter of hard and fast rules, but of weighing risks and making your own decision. In the same way, discuss the safety of over-the-counter medicines (such as pain-killers) with the pharmacist before buying them.

Aspirin

Pain-killers

Risks you can Choose to Avoid

- Smoking and breathing in other people's cigarette fumes.
- X-rays.
- All unnecessary medication.
- Heavy alcohol consumption.
- Illegal mood-changing drugs; for example, crack, heroin, cocaine, and marijuana.
- Raw and lightly cooked eggs – risk of salmonella poisoning.
- Soft cheeses and pâtés – risk of listeriosis.
- Contact with soiled cat litter or dog feces – risk of toxoplasmosis.
- Poisonous chemicals in household products; for example, paints, and wood preservatives such as creosote.
- Fumes from solvents; for example, cleaning fluids and adhesives.

Alcohol

"We moved during my pregnancy, and the garden fence needed treating with wood preservative. I knew some kinds were poisonous, so we made sure we bought a brand that was non-toxic."

"I enjoy walking in the country, but in my sixth month there was a helicopter spraying crops with what I suppose was pesticide, and I worried that it had damaged the baby. I went on worrying for another 18 weeks until she was born. I held her in my arms and wept with relief, because she was perfect."

"My doctor explained that the drugs I was taking to control my epilepsy could cause harelip and cleft palate, or even a heart malformation, in the baby. But she also told me that if I had seizures, they could cut off the baby's oxygen supply. So I had to balance the risk of having seizures against the risk of the drugs. I decided to continue with the medication."

GIVING UP SMOKING

If you smoke cigarettes, the single most caring thing you can do for your unborn baby is to give them up. Apart from the harm it does you – increasing your chance of a stroke or lung cancer – smoking may reduce the amount of oxygen available to your baby, stunt growth, constrict blood vessels, and lead to premature birth. If you decide to stop, make a ceremony of smoking your very last cigarette, and team up with someone else who is also quitting. People who have been used to having a cigarette in their hands say that it helps if they can do something that keeps their hands occupied in some other way, too.

If you feel it is impossible to give up cigarettes, there are two things you can do: cut down the number you smoke, and smoke only the first half of each one, throwing the rest away.

Indigestion tablets

~ WEIGHING RISKS ~

There is no such thing as a risk-free pregnancy, but don't let ideas of risk dominate your pregnancy. Every decision you make – even the simplest, such as whether to cross the street – entails making a choice. Every choice involves some risk. In pregnancy, weighing risks is especially complicated because you are thinking about at least two people – yourself and your baby – and probably about others, too: your partner, your older child, your parents, and your boss, for example. You need to be able to assess the risks and come to decisions in terms of your own life and the way you live it, how you feel, and the things that are important to you.

~ CREATING A SAFER ENVIRONMENT ~

To some extent your health, and that of your unborn baby, is in your hands. You can care for yourself well, eat the right foods, see that you get rest, and protect yourself and your baby from harmful chemicals as far as possible.

In nurturing yourself, you nurture your baby. Yet a pregnant woman's health is not only a matter of the choices she makes personally. It is affected also by the kind of society in which she lives, and by global events, such as war, famine, and the exploitation and destruction of the natural environment.

The damaging effects of human behavior on a large scale are issues of social policy and political change. Now is the time when you may decide to join consumer organizations and other pressure groups, and work towards making the world a safer and healthier place in which to live, so that all children can grow up in a safe environment.

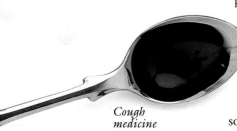

Cough medicine

SPECIAL TESTS

A VARIETY OF PRENATAL TESTS are offered that can reveal certain abnormalities in the baby. It may be taken for granted that, if a test reveals a handicap, you are sure to want a termination, but you do not have to agree to this. You may need time to sort out your thoughts, to discuss it with your partner and caregivers, and to find out more about the handicap before coming to a decision. Some women refuse these tests because they do not believe in terminating a pregnancy. Some want an abortion as soon as possible if the test proves positive. Others want to continue the pregnancy in the knowledge that the baby will die anyway, or are prepared to bear and cherish the handicapped child. Whatever the outcome, it should be your decision, not one made for you by doctors.

Getting the Results

- It may take four weeks or more for the results of an amniocentesis to come through.
- No test currently in use can guarantee a perfect baby.
- If a baby is revealed to have spina bifida (malformation of the spinal cord) or Down syndrome, no one can tell how badly it will be affected.
- Amniocentesis reveals the sex of the baby. You may or may not want to know what this is. Some people think it unwise for women to know, since they could be put under pressure to terminate a baby of the "wrong" sex.

I accept that there's a slight risk of miscarriage, but in my mind that weighs nothing against having a Down baby and the years of bringing up a handicapped child. I'm 40, and I wouldn't even consider getting pregnant unless these tests were available.

~ ALPHAFETA PROTEIN TEST (AFP) ~
This can reveal the possibility of a neural tube defect. The most common of these defects is spina bifida, when the baby's spinal cord is malformed. AFP is a simple, but very imprecise, test that measures protein in your blood. If you are having twins, or if your dates are not accurate, the protein level tends to be higher than usual. If AFP screening shows that there is an increased chance of the baby having a neural tube defect, you are offered an appointment for an amniocentesis.

~ AMNIOCENTESIS ~
Amniocentesis is usually done at 16 or 17 weeks, although it can be done earlier. It tests for Down syndrome and other genetic handicaps. Guided by ultrasound, and with a local anesthetic, a long needle is inserted through your abdominal wall and uterus to take a sample of amniotic fluid. The cells in the fluid are then grown in a culture. After the test, you may have some leakage of the amniotic fluid in which the baby is lying. There is a one per cent risk that amniocentesis will result in a miscarriage, and double the risk that the baby will have unexplained breathing problems at birth. About three per cent of tests fail to produce results the first time, so after some weeks the test is offered again.

AMNIOCENTESIS
Although the needle looks very close, the baby moves away as it is introduced.

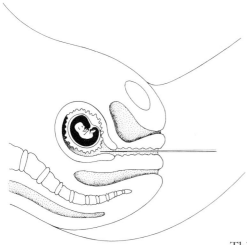

CHORIONIC VILLUS SAMPLING
The needle used to collect a sample of chorionic villi is guided by means of ultrasound.

" *If I were to have a handicapped baby, I'd be very sad, of course, but I couldn't agree to abort a baby because it was less than perfect, physically or mentally. So these tests are out of the question as far as I'm concerned.*"

"*I realized I'd had a blood test, but I didn't understand what for. Then I got a letter out of the blue, the day before we were supposed to be going on vacation, telling me that I had to have amniocentesis. I called and they advised me to cancel the flight tickets. It was terrifying! Then, when I had the amniocentesis, they couldn't find anything wrong. But it affected the whole of the rest of my pregnancy and I couldn't stop worrying.*"

"*At last I got the results. It wasn't spina bifida. I was so happy I cried for joy and spent the whole day phoning everyone I knew to tell them the good news.* "

~ CHORIONIC VILLUS SAMPLING (CVS) ~

This can be done as early as six weeks, which is why many people prefer it to amniocentesis if it is available. It tests for Down syndrome and other chromosome abnormalities. Chorionic villi, which look like tiny roots (see the photograph on page 41), will later form part of the placenta. They grow from the same fertilized cell as the baby, so they can provide clues about cells in the fetus. The biopsy is done through your vagina and cervix. A sample of cells is sucked out with a needle through a plastic tube and examined under a microscope. Unfortunately, research shows that there is a higher rate of miscarriage after CVS than after amniocentesis.

~ NUCHAL TRANSPARENCY TEST ~

This is a scan at 10–14 weeks to measure fluid at the back of the baby's neck. If there is a lot of fluid, there may be a chromosomal abnormality, such as Down syndrome. This test can be followed by amniocentesis. A scan at this time can also reveal other major fetal abnormalities.

UNDERSTANDING THE TESTS

Q   What questions do you want to ask your caregivers about the AFP test, amniocentesis, Nuchal screening, and CVS?

_____

_____

_____

_____

_____

_____

_____

TODAY'S DATE _____

AT WORK

ORKING OUTSIDE YOUR HOME does not generally make pregnancy and birth more difficult. It is often forgotten that occupational stress, heavy lifting, and toxic chemicals are problems just as much for women whose home and family are their work, as they are for those who go out to work in offices, laboratories, hospitals, or factories.

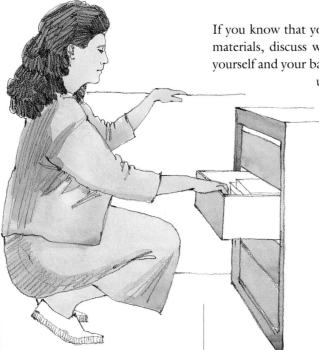

AVOIDING BACK STRAIN
Furniture is rarely designed with pregnant women in mind. Rather than stooping, squat down to reach low drawers.

" *They were very considerate at work. From six to 12 weeks I had bad nausea with bouts of vomiting on and off all day. I worked from home and could pace myself without being under pressure from anyone else.* "

~ MINIMIZING RISKS ~

If you know that you work in an unsafe environment or with hazardous materials, discuss with your doctor how you can minimize the risks to yourself and your baby. Your health and safety officer, company nurse, or union representative may be able to help, too. You should not have to work where other people are smoking, for example, as passive smoking cuts down the oxygen available to the baby through your bloodstream. Moving to a position beside an open window, or simply putting a fan on your desk, may reduce the effect of other people's smoking. But a definite no-smoking policy is much better.

~ KNOWING YOUR RIGHTS ~

Your own colleagues may be supportive, but some pregnant women meet an anti-baby attitude. They go back to work at the end of their maternity leave to discover that someone else has taken over their desk, or that they have been demoted. So know your legal rights, terms of employment, and conditions of maternity leave and pay.

TAKING A BREAK

If you have definitely decided to go back to work soon after the baby is born, it is a good idea to plan a vacation in mid-pregnancy if you can. At this stage you are likely to be feeling fit, and it will be your last opportunity for a real rest. It may give your energy a welcome boost, too, and fill you with added zest for the time after the birth.

Your maternity leave can start up to 11 weeks before the week the baby is due, but unless you have an unforeseen complication such as high blood pressure, you may want to go on working for as long as possible. After the birth, you may need to return to your job within 12 weeks in order to protect your employment rights. Check with your company.

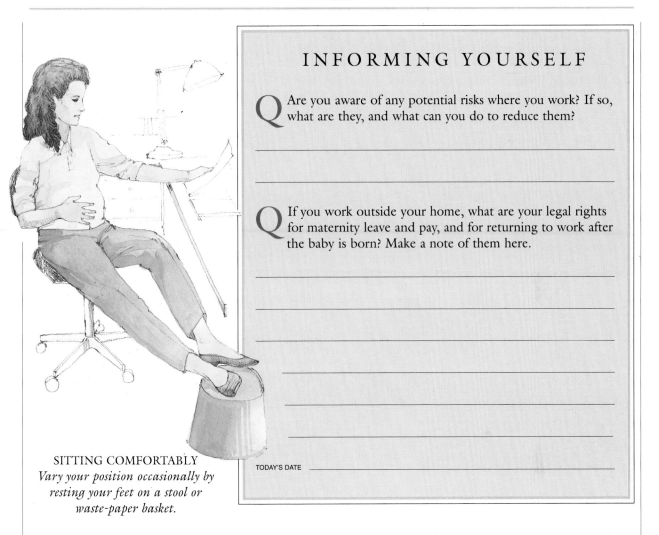

INFORMING YOURSELF

Q Are you aware of any potential risks where you work? If so, what are they, and what can you do to reduce them?

_____

_____

Q If you work outside your home, what are your legal rights for maternity leave and pay, and for returning to work after the baby is born? Make a note of them here.

_____

_____

_____

_____

_____

_____

TODAY'S DATE _____

SITTING COMFORTABLY
Vary your position occasionally by resting your feet on a stool or waste-paper basket.

~ GOING BACK TO WORK ~

If you are at home and plan to go back to work, think about how you can keep up-to-date with developments in your field, and stay in touch with colleagues. You may be able to negotiate a return to work part-time, to work flexible hours, or to do all or part of your job at home after the baby is born. For some jobs, telephones, fax machines, computers, and modems make working at home more feasible than it used to be. Whatever you decide, you will need good childcare. Where workplace on-site day care is not provided, women can sometimes get together to lobby for on-the-spot, high-quality childcare.

For the first months of your baby's life, and possibly longer, you will be working on night shift as well as during the day, so plan not to do too much too soon. Try to make time for an evening nap, or have someone bring you supper in bed. Flexible planning ahead for your working life with a baby, and getting a support network of other people who are willing to help you, are vital at this stage.

" My boss was happy for me to wait and see how life with the baby turned out to be before I made any decisions about when I would go back to work. I know of women in other firms who've been under pressure to decide a long time in advance, and they've felt awful if they've changed their minds later."

"A group of us is campaigning to have good, inexpensive childcare, more flexible working hours, and equal training and promotion opportunities."

Weeks 13 *to* 16

BY 16 WEEKS your metabolism has adjusted to pregnancy. The fatigue and nausea of the first weeks is likely to have vanished. Your uterus is the size of a large grapefruit. Its muscular wall is thick and strong, and starts to be stretched and thinned out. Think now of what you want most for your baby. All mothers have dreams for their children. We want them to be healthy and hope for a world in which they can grow up safely. Take time to get in touch with your feelings. Close your eyes and visualize the baby inside you. Focus on how your body is nurturing your baby.

Body Facts

• Your heart is beating stronger and faster to pump the increased quantity of blood around your body into the placenta.

• There are more blood vessels in your vagina, which becomes dark and soft, like crimson velvet.

• The thyroid gland in your neck has enlarged to up to twice its usual size, so you may find tight collars uncomfortable.

• Food takes longer to digest. The stomach of a woman who is not pregnant empties within 50 minutes. When you are pregnant, it takes 130 minutes.

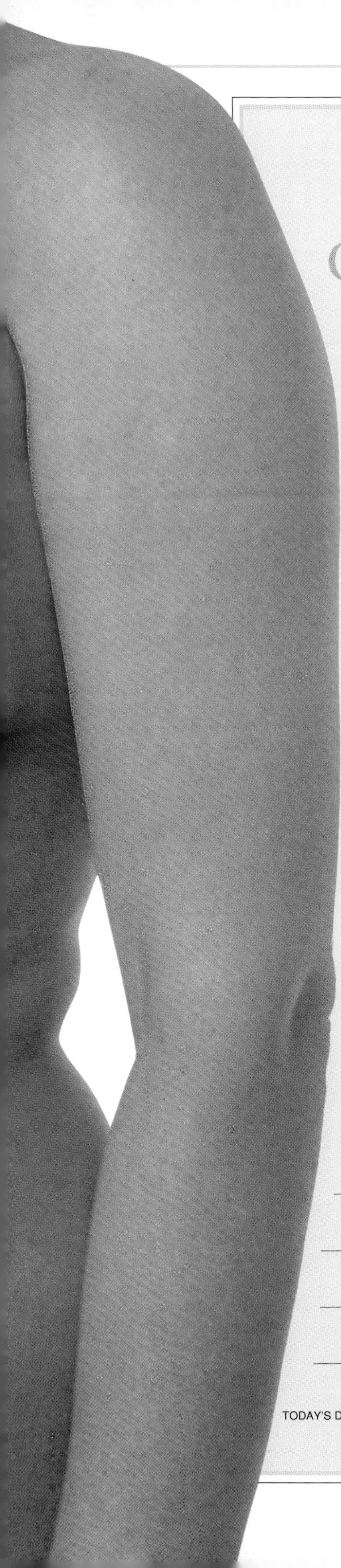

HOPES FOR YOUR BABY

Q If you could have three wishes for your baby, what would they be?

_____
_____
_____
_____
_____
_____
_____
_____
_____
_____
_____
_____
_____
_____
_____
_____
_____
_____
_____
_____
_____

TODAY'S DATE _____

Week 13   MONTH / DAY / YEAR

S
M
T
W
T
F
S

Week 14   MONTH / DAY / YEAR

S
M
T
W
T
F
S

Week 15   MONTH / DAY / YEAR

S
M
T
W
T
F
S

Week 16   MONTH / DAY / YEAR

S
M
T
W
T
F
S

HOW YOUR BABY IS GROWING

BY 16 WEEKS the main organs of the baby's body are formed. The bag of waters – the membranes – and the placenta inside it, together sustain the baby's life inside your uterus, as a space capsule provides everything that an astronaut needs.

The bag of waters cushions the baby from bumps, keeps it at a constant warm temperature, enables it to exercise its limbs and move freely, and provides liquid for it to practice swallowing. When you are in labor, the unbroken bag of waters helps your cervix open by producing hydrostatic pressure against it. The fluid contained in the bag is salt water, and so all the time the baby is inside you it is like a sea creature.

The baby turns somersaults, although you probably will not feel these movements until 18 or 20 weeks. It can turn its head, open its mouth, and move its chest and abdomen up and down as if breathing deeply. It can suck and swallow already, and may get hiccups. It yawns and stretches, and can raise its eyebrows and pucker up its forehead in a frown.

Feathery projections into the wall of the uterus are formed by chorionic villi.

The water inside the bubble of membranes is always warm and fresh. It replenishes itself completely every six hours.

Did You Know

• The baby can't get too hot or cold, partly because you regulate your own temperature by sweating if you are hot and shivering if you are cold. The fluid, membranes, muscular wall of the uterus, and your fat and skin also keep the baby warm. But if you get extremely hot, as in a sauna, your circulatory system is affected and you may get palpitations. This is not good for either the baby or you, so avoid high temperatures.

The baby weighs around 2 oz (60 g) and is 2 1/4 in (8 cm) from crown to rump, about the size of a duck egg.

The cord is soft like wet spaghetti, but much stronger. However much the baby bounces around, it rarely gets tangled.

THE PLACENTA

The blood that supplies oxygen to the baby's tissues from the air you breathe, and nutrients from the food you eat, flows through a fine membrane into the placenta. From there the oxygen and nutrients pass into the baby.

The placenta looks like a large piece of raw liver, and is fully formed by the twelfth week of pregnancy. Its branching blood vessels are the tree of life for your unborn baby. By the end of pregnancy it usually measures 7–8 in (17.5–20 cm) across – about the size of a dessert plate. It is approximately one-sixth of the baby's weight, and is the thickness of your thumb in the middle, but thinner around the edge.

The placenta develops from the outer covering of the fertilized cell cluster, and is made up of tiny, finger-like projections called chorionic villi that are grouped in lobes. These branch out in the lining of your uterus, as a tree is rooted in the earth. The baby's umbilical cord is usually attached to the center of the placenta.

Oxygenated blood is pumped through the vein in the cord into the baby's circulation. The blood from which oxygen has been extracted comes back through the arteries in the baby's cord to the placenta. The baby's waste products are filtered through the placenta into your bloodstream so that you can excrete them. The placenta is also a barrier against some infections, such as pneumonia and tuberculosis, and it manufactures hormones to maintain the pregnancy.

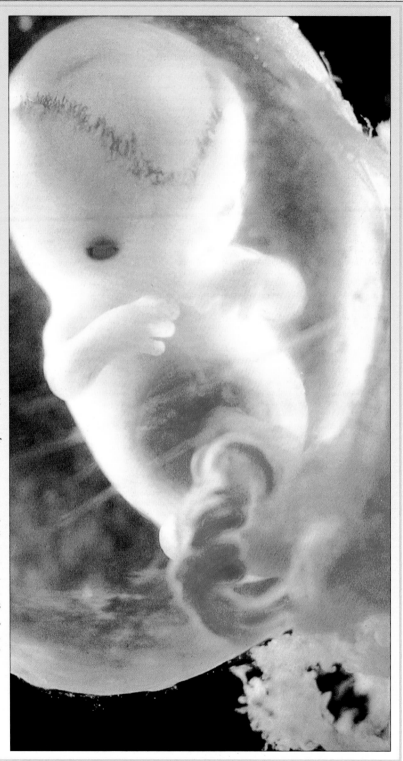

LIFE-SUPPORT SYSTEM
The placenta of this ten-week old fetus lies in the right-hand corner, next to the bag of waters.

KEEPING FIT

GENTLE EXERCISE IN PREGNANCY makes you feel good, improves circulation, and keeps you healthy. Regular exercise tones your muscles and keeps you supple. Swimming and cycling are especially good because your body is supported. A half-hour walk once a day – especially if you can take it in the countryside or in a park – is invigorating. Do some of the exercises on these pages daily. Put on your favorite music and relax. Taking time for yourself like this will help you feel refreshed, and get your body into good condition for labor.

~ ADJUSTING TO CHANGE ~

During pregnancy, the way you move every day is as important as any special exercises you do (*see* pages 56–57). Your body is heavier, weight distribution alters, your center of gravity changes, and there is increased joint movement in your pelvis. This pelvic rocking exercise tones your back and abdominal muscles, and helps your body adjust to these changes.

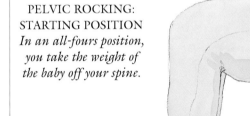

PELVIC ROCKING:
STARTING POSITION
In an all-fours position, you take the weight of the baby off your spine.

Helping Your Body Loosen

• All movement should be smooth and rhythmic.
• Continue breathing as you move. Don't hold your breath.
• Warm up before vigorous exercise, and relax afterwards.
• Avoid strenuous twisting and jerky movements.
• Avoid exercises – such as sit-ups and double leg lifting – that are a strain on abdominal and back muscles, and those that keep you on your back for any length of time.
• Pain is a signal to stop, or ease up on, an exercise.

~ TONING EXERCISES ~

You can do this exercise in an all-fours position as shown here, or lying on your back with your head and shoulders well supported (*see* page 57). Start with your back straight, knees and hands well apart, and head raised. Let your head drop, and press the small of your back up. Then raise your head and flatten your back. Repeat eight to ten times.

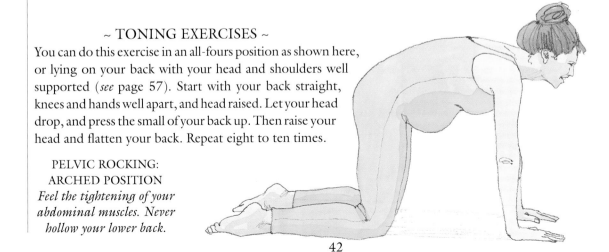

PELVIC ROCKING:
ARCHED POSITION
Feel the tightening of your abdominal muscles. Never hollow your lower back.

~ STRETCHING AND OPENING EXERCISES ~

To feel the stretch on the muscles of your inner thighs, and build up a sense of your body opening, stand with your feet hip-width apart. Hold on to the back of a chair for support and bend your knees. Lower your body as far as is comfortable, keeping your back straight, then stand up smoothly and slowly. You can increase the stretch for your inner thigh muscles by doing this exercise standing on the balls of your feet, with your ankles together and your heels raised off the floor.

Another good stretching and opening exercise that you can do with a partner is the one illustrated on pages 44 and 45. Stand facing each other with your feet wide apart and heels flat on the ground. Hold each other's arms at the wrist to make a counterbalance when you bend. Gently lower to a squat, keeping your back straight. Hold the position for a few seconds, then stand up slowly. Repeat to feel the stretch to your inner thighs.

~ MINIMIZING BACK STRAIN ~

Kneel forward with knees wide apart, leaning on your elbows. You can read or listen to music like this. In forward-leaning and all-fours positions, be careful not to let your lower back cave in, as this can cause back strain. When your spine is straight, the baby is supported by the sling of your abdominal muscles instead of pulling on those in your back.

~ EXERCISING IN WATER ~

To tone abdominal muscles, float in a swimming pool with your back against the pool-side, and arms extended along the top. Bending your knees, raise your legs to a right-angle with your body, then lower them to the bottom again. Brisk walking in the pool is good, too.

The women in the class were at least ten years younger than me, and very agile. I couldn't hold a squat for more than a few seconds and thought: I'm not going to be able to give birth to this baby. Now I'm doing gentle exercises in kneeling or half-kneeling positions, and exercising in water, too. I feel much more confident and positive about my body.

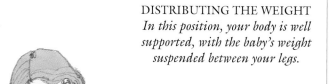
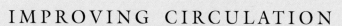
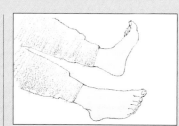

DISTRIBUTING THE WEIGHT
In this position, your body is well supported, with the baby's weight suspended between your legs.

I really enjoyed exercising in pregnancy. As I got bigger, I could roll my pelvis in a very satisfying way, and it felt good to do large, slow, sensuous movements."

"The only thing that reduced my backache was if I polished the floor on my hands and knees!"

"I don't usually do exercises. But they're a great way to keep in touch with changes in your body in pregnancy.

IMPROVING CIRCULATION

Sit in an easy chair with your legs straight out in front, ankles and knees relaxed. Place one heel on the floor, and extend your toes up and back towards you. Make circles with your big toe, first one way, then the other. Feel your calf muscles stretch and relax. Do this six times, then change to the other foot.

This foot exercise helps circulation, and is comfortable if you have swollen ankles.

THINKING ABOUT CLASSES

CHILDBIRTH CLASSES, run by the hospital, the birth center midwives, or by an independent childbirth organization, usually start at six or seven months and take place every week, although in some areas there are "early-bird" groups before this. Couples' classes are increasingly popular, but there are also groups for women only, and others are a mix of the two. Because styles of teaching vary, shop around to find classes that suit you best before signing up for a course.

Checklist

Good childbirth classes include:

• Information about making choices between alternatives, and negotiating the kind of care and birth place you want.
• Practicing relaxation.
• Breathing for labor.
• Rehearsal for how your partner can help you.
• Practicing different positions and movements for labor.
• Discussion of feelings before and after birth.
• The emotional as well as physical processes of birth.
• Discussion of breastfeeding, and how new babies behave.

~ MAKING A DECISION ~

Find out when classes take place (daytime or evening), who teaches them (usually a midwife, registered nurse, childbirth educator, or yoga instructor), whether or not partners can go, and what the classes include. Compare what is available with the suggestions in the checklist before you decide.

~ SHARING EXPERIENCES ~

Getting together with other women and couples, and sharing how you feel is helpful. You may make some good friends in classes, and can plan to meet regularly after your babies are born, too. A new mother encounters many challenges which can be overwhelming if she has to deal with them alone.

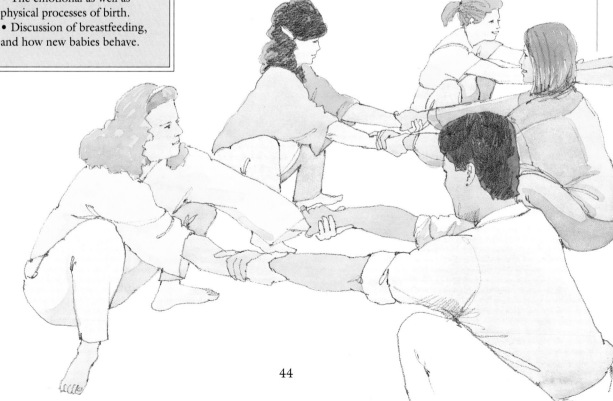

**These classes are good because I want to have a natural birth and I'm learning to open my body, and yet the instructor also goes into detail about what happens when things aren't straightforward, how you can help yourself, and how the people looking after you can help you.**

"I'm glad Michael's coming with me. At first he said he wasn't thrilled about rolling around on the floor, grunting and groaning with a lot of pregnant women. But all kinds of things are discussed, like good nutrition, for example, that he's never had a clue about, and sex in pregnancy and after the baby comes. He's gotten really interested, and lost all his self-consciousness, and made friends with some of the other men."

"The classes are great! Anne and I talk about the ideas that were aired all the way home in the car. It's not like a formal lecture and then a question-and-answer session. The group makes the classes, and we all discuss what we want and explore different topics. The teacher is a resource, a facilitator, and she's completely open to other people's ideas.

EXPLORING MOVEMENT
In childbirth classes you practice movements to tone your muscles and help you deal with any pregnancy discomforts, and learn how to open your pelvis for the birth. Working together, you gain confidence to handle the stress of labor.

YOUR CHOICE OF CLASSES

Q What kind of childbirth classes have you decided on?

_____

_____

Q Why did you choose these particular classes?

_____

_____

Q When do your classes start?

_____

Q Who teaches the classes?

_____

Q Can partners come to all or some of the classes?

_____

_____

Q What books does your childbirth educator suggest as useful reading?

_____

_____

_____

_____

_____

_____

TODAY'S DATE _____

HAVING A SCAN

A N ULTRASOUND SCAN shows the size and shape of a hidden solid object by means of high-frequency sound waves, which are inaudible to the adult ear. The sound waves are bounced off the object, producing echoes that are then changed into an image on a television screen. Ultrasound is used routinely in many countries – including the U.S. – at about the sixteenth week of pregnancy to assess the baby's size, and sometimes again in later pregnancy to reveal how the baby is lying in the uterus. At 16 weeks you can see the whole baby on the scan. Later in pregnancy only part of the baby's body is visible. A scan can diagnose twins and some genetic abnormalities, and may show the sex of your baby and where the placenta is lying. It can also determine whether the fetal heart is beating, if the woman thinks she is having a miscarriage.

SEEING YOUR BABY *Having a scan may be exciting, when you see the baby moving inside you.*

~ QUESTIONS OF SAFETY ~

Before ultrasound was invented, X-rays were used to find out what was happening in the uterus. Now it is known that these are dangerous, and that they can cause childhood cancer. Ultrasound appears to be much safer than X-rays, but no long-term follow-up studies of babies who have had scans are being done. Because we do not yet know enough about possible effects, ultrasound should be used only when it provides useful information and will make a difference to the kind of care you need during pregnancy or at the time of birth. You can refuse a scan if you do not want one.

~ GETTING THE MOST FROM A SCAN ~

If you have an ultrasound scan, you may find that it helps to have your partner or a friend with you. You can ask the radiographer, doctor or midwife to explain everything that is happening, and to interpret the image that you see on the screen.

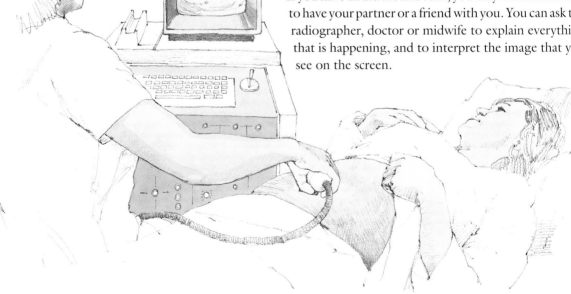

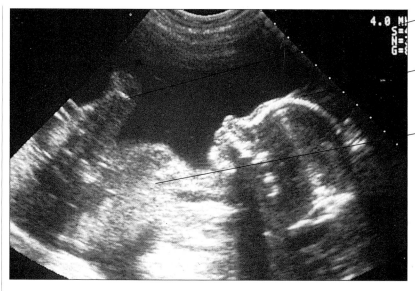

The baby's limbs may be visible, with stubby hands and feet.

The baby's head is oval. The forehead is broad and flat, and the nose snubbed.

The chest and abdomen are rounded.

UNDERSTANDING THE IMAGE
The image on the screen is like a hazy drawing. You can ask for the different parts of the baby to be shown. The latest development is 3-D ultrasound, which gives a clearer image.

"It was all conducted in silence and they wouldn't let me see the screen. I asked if everything was all right and the radiographer said she wasn't allowed to say, I must ask my own doctor. But I didn't have an appointment with him till a week after. I hated the whole thing."

"It was amazing to see that little thing wiggling around, nodding its head and sucking its thumb – and at one point it looked as if it was waving. They took a Polaroid photo of it that I keep under my pillow."

"I decided not to have a scan. I was certain of my dates, so we wouldn't have learned anything about that. I know the baby usually moves around and its heart speeds up when a scan is done, so maybe it doesn't like it. I couldn't see the point of a scan, so I said no.

PREPARING FOR A SCAN

Q What questions do you want to ask your doctor or midwife *before* you have a scan?

Q What information do you want the radiographer, doctor or midwife to give you if you have a scan?

TODAY'S DATE

WHAT IF IT'S TWINS?

By NOW YOU HAVE probably got over the shock of expecting twins. Although it is exciting, a multiple pregnancy is harder work and more tiring for a woman's body. The strain on muscles, bones, and joints is often greater and you may need extra rest and nutrition.

~ LOOKING AHEAD ~

If you are having more than one baby, there is a greater chance that your pregnancy and birth may be less straightforward. Because of this doctors automatically consider you to be "at risk," and often take it for granted that women will agree to induction of labor and an epidural, or planned Cesarean section. Getting what you want in childbirth therefore may be more difficult. There are sometimes good reasons why interventions would help – for example, because the first baby is lying in an awkward position – but you still have a right to all the information you need to make a decision.

Twins are often born two or three weeks early and may be smaller than single babies. You will need practical help then so that you have time with your babies.

REVISING YOUR BIRTH CHOICES

Q Now that you know you are expecting more than one baby, do you wish to change any of the choices you made for the birth and recorded on pages 16–17?

_____

_____

_____

_____

TODAY'S DATE _____

SHARING RESPONSIBILITY
Your partner's help can prevent you feeling trapped with unending work, and give you both time to enjoy your babies.

“ *After I'd got over the first shock I'm starting to enjoy it. I feel special. I'm looking after myself extra carefully because I want to give them the best start in life, and be in peak condition myself.* ”

HOW TWINS ARE FORMED

There are two ways in which twins develop. In the first, only one egg is produced and fertilized but splits into two complete cell cultures. In this case identical twins start to grow. In the second way, two or more ripe eggs are produced at the same time by either one or both ovaries. (If you have taken fertility drugs, even more may ripen.) In this case, sperm may join with more than one egg. Twins formed in this way are called fraternal twins and are no more alike than any other children in the family.

At the hospital they tend to treat me as if the pregnancy is an abnormal medical condition, but it's all going well and I feel great.

IDENTICAL TWINS

Identical twins are monozygotic, or one-egg, twins. They are rarer than fraternal twins. Only one-third of all twins are identical, half of them girl-pairs and half of them boy-pairs. Most have separate bubbles of amniotic fluid. Occasionally identical twins form after the membrane has developed, at about 14 days, and then they are inside the same bubble.

They nearly always share a placenta. Although identical twins resemble each other closely, are always the same sex, and may be mirror images of each other, it is important for each twin to be allowed to grow and develop as an individual, not as just half of a pair.

Identical (one-egg) twins

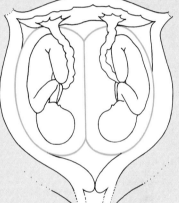

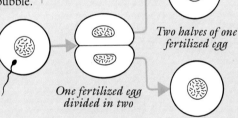

One egg

One sperm

Two halves of one fertilized egg

One fertilized egg divided in two

FRATERNAL TWINS

Fraternal twins are dizygotic, or two-egg, twins. Half of all fraternal twins will be a boy–girl pair, a quarter both boys, and a quarter both girls. They have two separate bubbles of amniotic fluid and two separate placentas, but sometimes they are lying so close together that the placentas fuse and look like one. Most fraternal twins grow from eggs fertilized at the same time, but occasionally the second egg is fertilized a couple of days later. Even then, both babies are often born within minutes of each other.

Fraternal (two-egg) twins

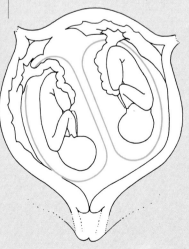

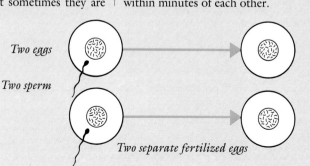

Two eggs

Two sperm

Two separate fertilized eggs

SPECIAL CARE PREGNANCIES

YOU MAY HAVE A PREGNANCY that is difficult because of an existing illness – diabetes, heart disease, severe asthma, or epilepsy, for example – or because one has developed during pregnancy. Even if your condition produces no complications at all, you may find that you are treated as high risk. Because of this, you will probably be advised to have your baby in a large hospital. You still have a right to information about alternatives, and to share in all the decisions made about you and your baby's care.

If you have a condition that needs special care, you experience the same joy and excitement at being pregnant, but probably have doubts as to how you will cope. Day-to-day support and understanding from someone close to you are vital.

~ WOMEN WITH DIABETES ~

If you are diabetic, your dietary needs change during pregnancy. This means that insulin requirements do, too. You are the expert in controlling your diabetes, so you can do much of your own glucose monitoring at home.

During pregnancy, you will be seen by a consultant who specializes in diabetes, as well as an obstetrician. Prenatal checks are usually twice a month until 32 weeks and weekly thereafter.

Babies of diabetic mothers are often larger, so you will probably have scans to monitor your baby's growth. This is to check that the baby doesn't get too big for a normal vaginal delivery. Labor may be induced when the baby is of a good size and maturity for birth even if not full term.

Most babies of diabetic mothers do not need to be separated from them after birth for special care, although some may need help with breathing.

~ WOMEN WITH DISABILITIES ~

Pregnancy is often an exciting and precious time for you because you discover that your body works in the same way as other women's. Any disability can make pregnancy tiring, and being a mother tends to be more exhausting even than for unimpaired women. You may need extra equipment for housework and dealing with the baby. Like many new mothers, you may find yourself at home for 24 hours a day. One really helpful thing is to be in touch with other women in similar situations, and to learn how they have coped.

CAREFUL CONTROL
Monitoring your glucose allows you to adjust your diet if necessary.

"*I am a pregnant woman who happens to have asthma, not an asthmatic who is pregnant!*"

"*When we said we were expecting a baby, you could see their faces, 'How on earth did that happen?' They really don't think disabled people have a normal sex life like everyone else.*"

Your biggest problem may be other people's attitudes, and their anxieties about how you will cope. What women with disabilities say themselves is that they want more than just admiration and being told how wonderful they are. They need practical help so that they can function as ordinary members of society, with emphasis on themselves as human beings, rather than on their disabilities.

~ DISABILITIES OF SIGHT AND HEARING ~

If you are blind or deaf, seek out a childbirth organization that can either offer classes that cater specifically for your needs, or where the teacher is flexible enough to adapt her teaching methods to you.

Because difficulty with hearing cannot be seen, people may not be aware of it, and may fail to realize that they are not communicating adequately. So writing a Birth Plan is important, to demonstrate that you are considering alternatives, and also to ensure that your caregivers know what you want.

> *The midwife advised me not to take Demerol because it makes you drowsy. That's the one thing I must not be if I'm to lip-read properly."*

> *"After I'd finished breastfeeding, my baby used to sleep in my arms. I remember how healing he'd been inside my body. He seemed to keep me so well, and continued to do so when I was holding him."*

> *"I need exercises I can do in a wheelchair, but no one's suggested any.*

WHAT HAPPENS IF YOU ARE RHESUS NEGATIVE

A Rhesus negative mother may have a Rhesus positive baby, unless she knows for certain that the baby's father is Rhesus negative too. If she bleeds during pregnancy or at the birth, some of the baby's positive blood may leak into her circulation. This seems like a foreign body to her immune system, and she may make antibodies.

It is very unusual for this to happen in a first pregnancy, but more likely in subsequent pregnancies. So a Rhesus negative mother is always given an injection of anti-D immunoglobulin (or Rhogam) – which is itself an antibody – after her first baby is born, and perhaps during her first pregnancy too. (She should also be given this after a miscarriage or termination.)

This "fools" the body into behaving as if it had already manufactured its own antibodies, so that it does not treat the next baby as an "invading alien".

A blood test will show if she has produced antibodies in a previous pregnancy. If she has, but was not given Rhogam then, she will need special care in any future pregnancy.

First pregnancy

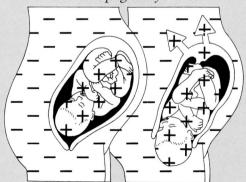

- Rh negative blood
+ Rh positive blood
▲ Rhesus antibodies

If a Rhesus negative woman bleeds in a first pregnancy, her immune system may make antibodies.

Subsequent pregnancies

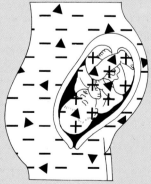

In subsequent pregnancies, these antibodies cross the placenta, and may harm a Rhesus positive baby.

Weeks 17 *to* 20

B Y 20 WEEKS there is a sense of having settled down into the pregnancy. The chance of miscarriage is much reduced, and you are beginning to adjust physically. Now is the time to start exercises in relaxation and body awareness in preparation for the birth. You may be lucky to find "early-bird" classes in your area, but most women have to do these exercises on their own.

Body Facts

• Your blood vessels may be more visible beneath your skin because your heart is now pumping 20 per cent extra blood through them.

• If you press your fingers in, you may be able to feel the top of your uterus a finger's width below your navel.

• Your uterus is no longer pear-shaped, but egg-shaped.

• You may have gained about 9 lb (4 kilos). This includes 10 oz (300 g) of baby, 6 oz (170 g) of placenta, and 12 oz (350 g) of amniotic fluid.

• Your breasts are larger, and the nipples and the area around them may be darker.

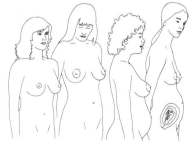

YOUR BODY IS UNIQUE *Even at the same stage of pregnancy, every woman's shape and size differs according to her height and build.*

❝ *I didn't understand how early in pregnancy breasts changed. I noticed that they were tender even before I knew I was pregnant. Then my bra was too tight. Now I've had to get a cup D size."*

"I don't feel especially pregnant. My waist is a bit thicker and there are little bumps around my nipples, but that's all. I lost weight at first because I was being sick, but now I'm putting it on again."

"There's a nice curve low in my abdomen that I think of already as 'baby.' My breasts have always been small, not a part of my body I've liked much. Now they've filled out and I'm rather pleased with my figure. ❞

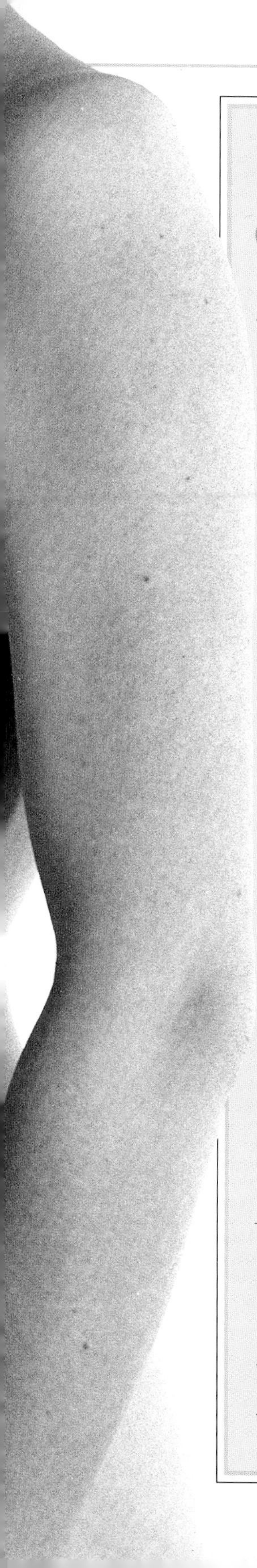

BODY CHANGES

Q Have your breasts grown larger or heavier?

_____

Q Are your breasts particularly tender or sensitive? Do they tingle?

_____

Q Is the circle around your nipples any darker?

_____

_____

Q Apart from breast changes, what other changes do you notice?

_____

_____

_____

Q What does your waist measure now?

_____

Q What is the measurement around your hips and bottom?

_____

Q Have you gained weight? If so, how much?

_____

TODAY'S DATE _____

Week 17   MONTH / DAY / YEAR

S
M
T
W
T
F
S

Week 18   MONTH / DAY / YEAR

S
M
T
W
T
F
S

Week 19   MONTH / DAY / YEAR

S
M
T
W
T
F
S

Week 20   MONTH / DAY / YEAR

S
M
T
W
T
F
S

HOW YOUR BABY IS GROWING

BY 20 WEEKS you start to feel the baby's movements. At first they are as faint as the swish of butterfly wings or darting fish. Then you feel knocks, rolls, bumps, and insistent kicking as the baby turns, twists, jumps and somersaults inside you. Often she moves especially energetically in the evenings.

The baby can move freely because she is lying in salt water, which gives her extra buoyancy, and because the muscular wall of your uterus is springy, allowing her to bounce around like a cork in a bowl of water. By pushing against the muscle with her feet and head, she exercises and tones developing muscles as she begins to orient herself in space. As she matures, the baby probably enjoys this feeling of tumbling around.

The head is large in proportion to the rest of the body. Fine hair is starting to grow.

The baby is now 5½ in (14 cm) from crown to rump. She weighs 7 oz (200 g), about the same as a large orange.

The baby sucks her thumb, practicing movements that she will need for feeding later on.

The baby still has plenty of room to move around freely in the uterus.

The wall of the uterus is springy, so the baby can push and exercise her limbs against it.

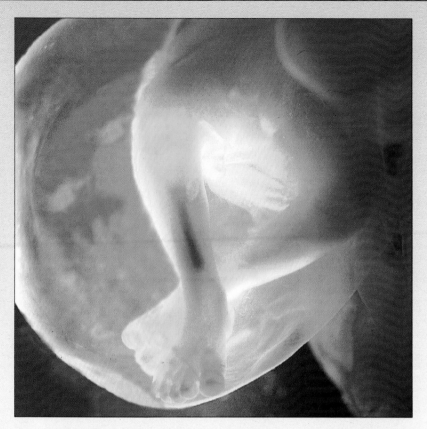

A GROWING AWARENESS
Now you start to feel the first kicks, and the baby becomes more of a real person in your mind.

"*I didn't recognize what it was at first. It was like something shifting around inside me. Then I realized that it was my baby! Now I'm waiting for it all the time, it's so exciting!*"

"*It went 'bump' right in the middle of a concert. The brass section was blaring and suddenly the baby leapt. I am sure it heard the music. It was the most incredible feeling!*"

Did You Know

- Some babies are much more active than others. This has nothing to do with whether it is a boy or a girl.
- You feel on average 9 out of every 10 movements, but this varies. Some women feel only 6 out of every 10 movements.
- A baby may spend up to 90% of its time moving, although the average is about 20%.
- Breathing movements increase from 0.5% of the time at 2 weeks to 6% at 19 weeks. Then, as the baby matures, breathing becomes more regular, although she can't breathe in air. This is like a rehearsal for the moments after birth.

~ WHEN DOES THE BABY MOVE? ~

Each baby tends to have its own characteristic rhythm of activity and moves most energetically at a particular time of the day. If you have been pregnant before, you may notice that this baby moves at different times from your first baby. You won't feel all the movements your baby makes – sucking, the fluttering of hands, and breathing movements are all too slight to notice.

A baby may be inactive for several hours at a time when she is probably sleeping. If you take sedatives, fetal movement is further reduced because the baby is sedated as well. If you drink alcohol heavily, the baby exercises her breathing muscles less often because alcohol depresses the nervous system, which controls breathing. If you smoke, shortage of oxygen causes the baby to make fewer breathing movements, too. Both alcohol and nicotine probably also interfere with the unborn baby's sleep patterns because they reduce oxygen in the bloodstream. When premature babies have been short of oxygen in the uterus, they tend to sleep badly.

If you have an ultrasound scan (*see* pages 46–47), the noise that you cannot hear (because the sound waves are at a frequency above the range audible to you) will wake up a healthy baby and stimulate her to activity. Her pulse-rate goes up, too.

MOVING WELL

A WOMAN OFTEN LEARNS for the first time in pregnancy that she cannot take her healthy body for granted. As she gets heavier, there may be aches and pains, most of which can be avoided by learning good body mechanics. When you are pregnant, you need to know how to use your body wisely, and the art of standing, walking, sitting, and lifting without straining.

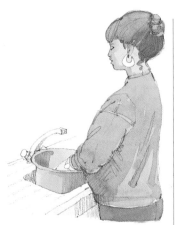

STANDING WELL
Tuck your bottom in. Stand on both feet with the weight spread equally, evenly balanced between heels and toes. Stretch tall, right up to the crown of your head. Drop your shoulders. Relax your knees.

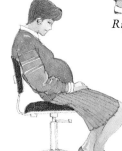

Right

Wrong

DOING DISHES
Standing in front of the sink, you should be able to place the palms of your hands flat on the bottom of the sink without stretching. If you can't, put a dishpan on top of another upside-down pan to raise your working height.

Right

Wrong

SITTING WELL
Sit well back in the chair with your back and thighs supported, legs slightly apart, feet flat on the floor.

“ *The worst thing is cleaning the tub. Leaning over gives me a backache – so now I always kneel, and it's much easier.*”

LIFTING THINGS FROM THE GROUND
Get close to the object. Squat down, bending your knees and keeping your back straight. Hold the object against your body, with elbows bent.

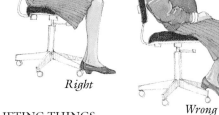

“*When I get up in the morning, I roll over on to all fours and maneuver off the bed that way. If I don't do that, I get a nagging ache low down in my back.*”

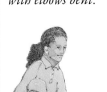

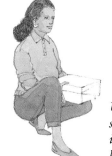

Using the muscles in your legs, straighten up slowly and smoothly into a standing position. Bend your knees, not your back.

LOADING AND UNLOADING A CAR TRUNK

If possible, get someone to maneuver heavy loads, such as groceries, into and out of a car trunk for you. Otherwise, learn how to deal with them yourself, safely and without straining.

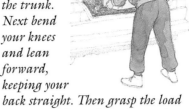

To load: *Stand with one hip (if you are of average height) or one thigh (if you are taller than average) against the edge of the trunk. With*

feet well apart, rest the load on the edge of the trunk. Next bend your knees and lean forward, keeping your back straight. Then grasp the load firmly and lift it into the trunk.

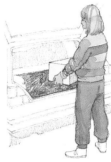

To unload: *Start in the same position as the last position of loading. Stand with one hip or thigh against the edge of the trunk.*

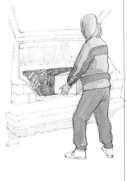

Bend your knees, and place both hands under the load. Bend your arms from the elbows to lift the load on to the edge of the trunk.

Bring the load against your body and straighten your legs. Use two hands for each bag to unload groceries.

TONING MUSCLES

You can prepare your body for changes in later pregnancy, and avoid or ease a backache, by toning muscles. Concentrate on your pelvic floor muscles which support the baby, your uterus, and all your abdominal organs, and those that support the muscles of your lower back and abdomen.

PELVIC ~ FLOOR MUSCLES ~

The muscles of the pelvic floor tighten when you stop a flow of urine. You can feel them if you slip a finger into your vagina and squeeze. Picture the figure eight of muscles around your vagina and urethra above, and your rectum below. Tighten these muscles so that the round shapes change to almond shapes. Hold them tightly for a few seconds. Then relax. Repeat five times. Finish the whole exercise with a tightening movement.

ABDOMINAL AND ~ LOWER BACK MUSCLES ~

Try doing the pelvic rock to music. Lie on your back with one or two pillows under your head and shoulders, legs comfortably apart, with knees bent and feet flat on the floor. Tilt your pelvis so that the small of your back presses against the floor. Then release the pressure. Repeat eight times. Rest. Then have another try.

CHOOSING ~ YOUR OWN ACTIVITY ~

Any activity that you enjoy, involving rhythmic movement with regular intervals for rest, will tone your body and increase your circulation, especially swimming and energetic walking. Physical tasks with a pleasurable working rhythm, such as mopping the floor, will tone muscles, too.

BECOMING A FATHER

MEN ARE OFTEN EXCITED ABOUT PREGNANCY because they feel it is proof of their masculinity and they become more self-confident. Sometimes you both have wanted a baby for a long time. Yet even then, approaching fatherhood also brings a sense of heavy responsibility, and a man may be anxious that his freedom will be curtailed. It helps to bring these conflicts out into the open and talk about them with your partner.

~ HOW YOUR PARTNER MAY FEEL ~

Some men switch off from pregnancy because they feel there is nothing they can do to help. They may be afraid to expose their vulnerability and caring feelings because they share the widespread male taboo on tenderness. Sometimes a man feels jealous of all the attention his partner is getting. Your partner may be scared of the enormous impending change in your life together, he may have deep, secret fears about birth, or perhaps worry that the baby will take love away from him.

~ TENSIONS IN YOUR RELATIONSHIP ~

Although there is often a new excitement and depth of tenderness in a couple's relationship, problems may come to the surface, too. They may have been there all the time, but they are made more obvious by the pregnancy since this is a major change in both your lives.

~ TALKING THINGS OVER ~

It is important to talk together about your feelings and not to get trapped in separate worlds. You are both becoming parents, and the transition is easier if there is understanding between you and an awareness of each other's feelings. It will probably help if you go together to the kind of childbirth classes where there is open discussion of feelings and relationships.

POSITIVE CHANGES
Pregnancy can add a new dimension to your relationship.

I've never thought of myself as a father. It's like growing up all of a sudden. In a funny way it makes me feel more equal to Dad – a man, not a boy.

~ PREPARING FOR THE BIRTH ~

Many fathers today are present at the birth of their children, but even if your partner is delighted about becoming a father, and you both want him to be there, he may still feel anxious, especially if you are having your first baby. It is distressing for anyone to be plunged into an experience for which he or she is unprepared. Explain to your partner what you want and how you feel so that he knows and understands what is going to happen. Discuss with him how he can help you during labor and birth.

John's worried for me because I'm 42 and he wants me to plan for a Cesarean section. I'd like it to be as natural as possible, so I need to help him to understand how I feel.

"Ours was a casual relationship before the baby started. We enjoyed each other, but we weren't committed. Finding out I was pregnant changed all that and we're doing more things together. Having a child makes you feel closer. You have a new time-scale."

"He doesn't want to talk about the baby. He's detached himself from it, and flings himself into his job. I feel alone."

"I know I'm supposed to be the strong shoulder she can lean on, but I don't always feel like that. At times I worry that the baby will be handicapped, but I can't talk about that because I'm meant to be supporting her."

"She's talking about the baby all dreamy-eyed and I'm worrying about the mortgage."

"I feel extraneous to everything that's happening to her. I've been to the doctor's office a couple of times and they say, 'Sit there!', and ignore me. She wants me to go along with her to discuss what she'd like when she goes into labor, and I'm going to have to be assertive and insist that they listen to us."

"The pregnancy doesn't feel real to me. I can't get excited about it. Maybe later on, when she shows more, I'll get into the spirit of it.

LOOKING AHEAD TOGETHER

Q Do you want your partner to be present at the birth?

_____

Q How does your partner feel about being at the birth?

_____

Q What plans are you making together so that your partner knows what to expect during labor?

_____

_____

_____

_____

Q What special help do you need from your partner during your pregnancy?

_____

_____

_____

Q What other things could you do together so that your partner understands your needs and can enjoy the birth?

_____

_____

_____

_____

_____

TODAY'S DATE _____

OTHER RELATIONSHIPS

WHEN A BABY IS BORN every relationship you have changes, however subtly. This is especially marked within the family and with people who are closest to you. Relationships with friends at work alter as you either become a mother like your colleagues, or somebody invisibly set apart from them because they don't have children. In the first few weeks of your baby's life you will be concentrating most on caring for her needs, so will have little time for other people.

FRESH PERSPECTIVES
Watching your parents with the baby, you see them in a different light. For a man who may not have taken time off to be with his own children, becoming a grandfather can bring unexpected pleasures.

~ YOU AND YOUR PARENTS ~

Your parents may be longing to become grandparents, or they may be indifferent, or not like the idea at all. They may find it difficult to accept that you are no longer their "child", or feel that they have suddenly become much older, or look forward excitedly to taking over the baby. Your relationship with your own mother often changes profoundly as you become a mother yourself. Talk together about how you both feel. In sharing an experience that was important for her, too, you may find a new friendship and understanding together.

~ PREPARING OLDER CHILDREN ~

You can help to prepare an older child for the baby now. Tell happy stories about when she was inside you and the exciting things that happened when she was born. Take her with you to the doctor's office. Ask the doctor or midwife to let her listen to her own heart with the stethoscope, and then listen to the baby's heartbeat. She will realize that the baby is not a doll curled up inside you, but a living person waiting to be born.

If you are moving her out of your bedroom, or from crib to bed, or if she is going to start at a play-group or nursery school, do this well before the birth, or she may take it as a sign of rejection.

~ CHILDREN'S CLASSES ~

Some childbirth educators run special classes for older siblings, or will take time out of a class to talk about what a baby can do or feel inside "mommy's belly," and to show how the baby is born, demonstrating with a life-size doll. They help children to understand that the new baby will not be able to play with them yet.

You may like to use the photographs and drawings in this book to talk about pregnancy and birth with your older child, too.

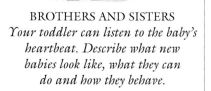

BROTHERS AND SISTERS
Your toddler can listen to the baby's heartbeat. Describe what new babies look like, what they can do and how they behave.

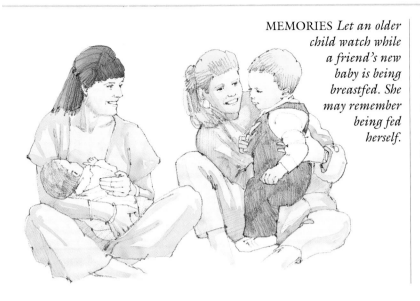

MEMORIES *Let an older child watch while a friend's new baby is being breastfed. She may remember being fed herself.*

" *The hospital had wonderful preparation classes for siblings. The woman who ran them dealt with feelings as well as facts – feeling left out in the cold, feeling anxious when the baby cries, feeling angry when the baby knocks over your Legos – that kind of thing. At the end of the course they all got 'big brother' or 'big sister' T-shirts."*

"I'd grown away from my parents. Then, with my pregnancy I got interested in what birth was like for my mother, and a new friendship is starting to develop out of that. "

HELPING YOUR CHILDREN TO ADJUST

Q How can you help your older children to understand your pregnancy and the birth of the new baby?

_____

_____

_____

_____

_____

_____

_____

_____

_____

_____

Q What ideas do you have for helping your older children to adjust to the new baby?

_____

_____

_____

_____

_____

_____

_____

_____

_____

TODAY'S DATE _____

IF YOU ARE ALONE

IF YOU ARE A SINGLE MOTHER you may be on your own because you chose to be so, or because you have no choice. Either way, it helps if there are other people with whom you can share the adventure of pregnancy. Having a birth partner – someone to whom you are close, and with whom you can relax easily – makes a great deal of difference to how you experience the birth.

~ LOOKING TO THE FUTURE ~

Now is the time to start building a good support network for after the baby is born, and get to know whom you can rely on for practical help. You will need high-quality childcare and, if you plan to return to a job outside home, flexible working arrangements. It isn't good for any mother to be isolated with a baby for hours on end. Meeting other people at a community center or mother-and-baby group – even just talking with other women at the playground – can help you to enjoy being a mother. The problems you may face, feeling that you have to carry total responsibility for your baby, are often shared by women who are not alone. Caring for your baby, and watching your child grow and develop, you may discover strengths, talents, and abilities you never knew you had.

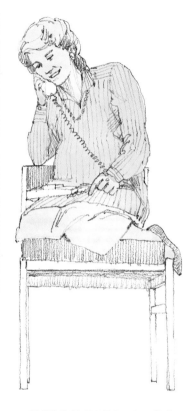

KEEPING IN TOUCH *It is especially important if you are alone to avoid being cut off from friends, and to have a circle of people who will support you.*

SHARING AND CARING *With a friend you can share some of the intense emotions of motherhood.*

“*I hid my pregnancy for as long as I could. Then my mother saw me in the bathtub. She was really good about it. Some of my school friends won't come near me. Maybe they think it's catching.*”

Getting Organized

- Get help with your finances if you need it.
- Find out about housing options.
- Check up on any social benefits to which you may be entitled.
- Register as early as you can for childbirth classes.
- Let your childbirth educator know you're on your own, so that she can give you the special help and support you need.

- Get to know other women in a similar position through organizations that are geared towards single parents.
- Find out about childcare facilities in your area and at work.
- Keep a checklist of organizations, agencies, friends, family, neighbors, and any other people you can call on for help, with their telephone numbers.

YOUR SUPPORT NETWORK

Q To whom do you turn for friendship and
support during your pregnancy?

_____

_____

_____

_____

Q Who will you ask to support you during
labor?

_____

_____

_____

Q Who will help you after the baby is born?

_____

_____

Q How can these people best support you
emotionally?

_____

_____

_____

_____

_____

TODAY'S DATE _____

Q How can these people help you in practical
ways?

_____

_____

_____

_____

_____

_____

_____

_____

_____

_____

_____

PLANNING AHEAD _Draw on other people's
experiences and enlist their help._

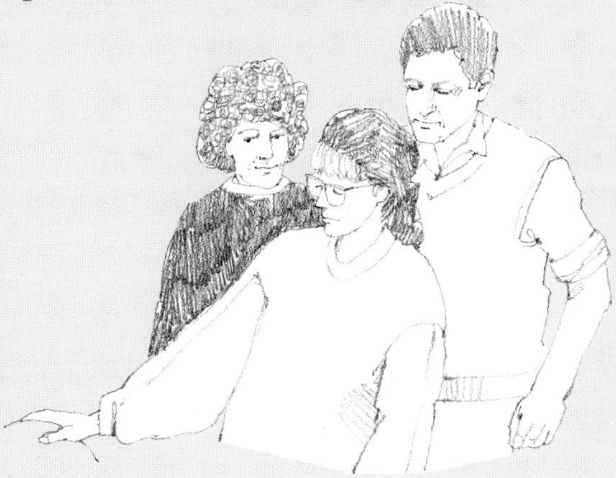

Weeks 21 *to* 24

By 24 WEEKS the top of your uterus is swelling just above your navel. You are probably gaining between half a pound (240 g) and a pound (480 g) a week. Now that the physical and emotional adjustments of early pregnancy are over, you may be feeling very good about yourself, and be fitter than ever before. Your eyes shine, hair is lustrous, and skin clear, and you walk with a spring in your step. If you lost interest in sex at the beginning of pregnancy, as many women do, it has now probably returned. When you make love, it is more comfortable if you explore positions where your partner's weight does not press down on you. Sex that is slow, gentle, and unhurried is the best kind for pregnancy. Knowing that the baby is growing inside you, and enjoying the ripe fullness of your body, may introduce for both of you new subtleties in your relationship, as well as intense pleasure.

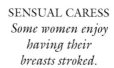

SENSUAL CARESS
*Some women enjoy
having their
breasts stroked.*

Body Facts

• Pregnancy changes your breathing. High levels of the hormone progesterone stimulate breathing so that more air is breathed in and out. When resting, you can breathe more deeply than you did before you were pregnant. To help yourself breathe well:
• See that your posture is good.
• Breathe slowly and fully down into your pelvis.
• As you breathe, focus on each complete, relaxed breath out, and you will find that the breath in will look after itself.

Sex is very exciting now because I don't have to think about contraception or worry about getting pregnant. I can be spontaneous.

"Our last baby was very premature, so now that it's coming up to the same time, we still make love but it doesn't involve penetration."

"I feel uncomfortable with my body. It's difficult to relax and make love, even though Peter loves the way it looks now.

PLANNING AHEAD

Q Looking ahead to the weeks after the birth, what plans are you making so that you have time and energy for your baby?

_____

_____

Q What help are you likely to need with everyday household tasks?

_____

_____

Q What help do you want to have with the baby during the day and at night?

_____

_____

Q What help would you like with your older child(ren)?

_____

_____

Q Is your partner going to help care for the baby?

_____

_____

Q How does your partner plan to get to know the baby?

_____

TODAY'S DATE _____

Week 21 MONTH / DAY / YEAR

S
M
T
W
T
F
St

Week 22 MONTH / DAY / YEAR

S
M
T
W
T
F
St

Week 23 MONTH / DAY / YEAR

S
M
T
W
T
F
S

Week 24 MONTH / DAY / YEAR

S
M
T
W
T
F
S

HOW YOUR BABY IS GROWING

BY 24 WEEKS the baby's organs of balance inside the ear have developed and are already of adult size. You may feel as if you have a jumping bean rolling around inside you as the baby balances himself head-down, then head-up, then sideways, before tumbling over again.

At the end of this period the eyes open. The baby has delicate eyelashes and eyebrows now. It isn't dark all the time inside the uterus, since bright sunlight and strong artificial light can filter through your abdominal wall, producing a rosy glow. Then, when you turn away from the light, the uterus is plunged into darkness again.

The baby can suck and sometimes sucks his thumb. Even at this early stage, he is learning to co-ordinate satisfying sucking and swallowing in readiness for feeding after birth.

The skin is red and very wrinkled as if it doesn't quite fit. It is so thin that the network of blood vessels shows through like delicate patterns on a crimson lampshade when the light is on.

Now, if your caregiver finds the right spot – and this may not be easy because the baby is moving around – the baby's heart can be heard not only with ultrasound, but with a stethoscope or a Pinard's trumpet-shaped fetal stethoscope. Its beat sounds like an old-fashioned watch ticking under a pillow. Sometimes the stethoscope picks up a soft, blowing sound, too. This uterine souffle is caused by the flow of blood through arteries in your uterus, and matches your own pulse-rate.

From the crown of his head to his rump, the baby measures approximately 8 in (20 cm) – about the length of a large man's hand from the wrist to the tip of the second finger.

Fingernails have formed now.

The baby can make a fist, and punches with it against the muscular uterine wall.

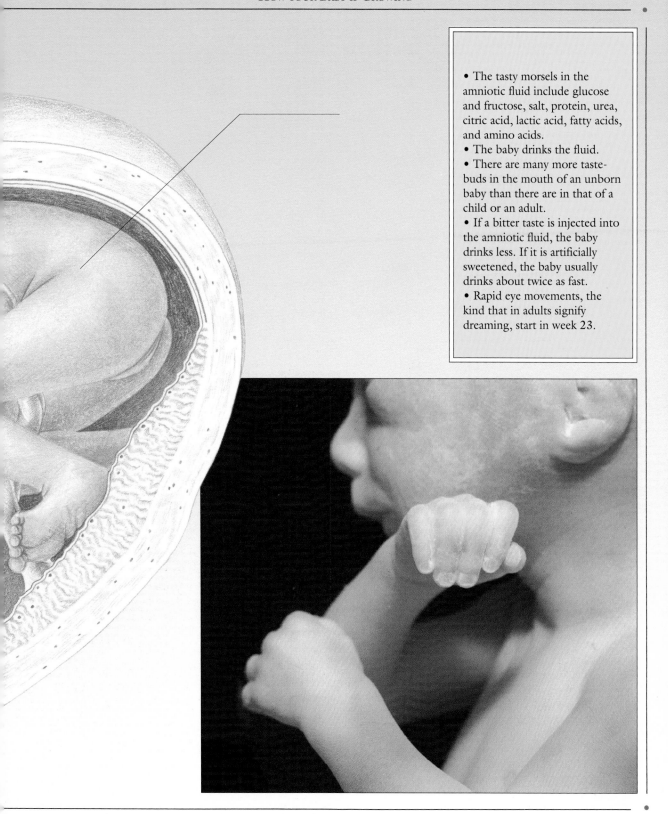

- The tasty morsels in the amniotic fluid include glucose and fructose, salt, protein, urea, citric acid, lactic acid, fatty acids, and amino acids.
- The baby drinks the fluid.
- There are many more taste-buds in the mouth of an unborn baby than there are in that of a child or an adult.
- If a bitter taste is injected into the amniotic fluid, the baby drinks less. If it is artificially sweetened, the baby usually drinks about twice as fast.
- Rapid eye movements, the kind that in adults signify dreaming, start in week 23.

YOUR FEELINGS

PREGNANCY IS A TIME of rapid and dramatic change, so it is not surprising that sometimes you may feel flooded by emotion. You grow as a person. Many women have a sense of being more complete – more whole – with the baby developing inside them. Yet pregnancy is also a period of adjustment: life is never going to be the same again and you may have many conflicting feelings.

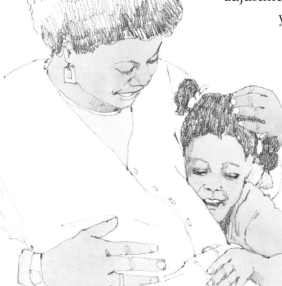

BEING IN TOUCH *Sharing the thrill of pregnancy creates a new bond between mother and child.*

~ TENDERNESS AND COMPASSION ~

You notice babies and feel tender about them. You may be very disturbed at seeing on television news programs children who are injured, maltreated or starving, and find that tears well up readily.

~ BEING MORE IN-TURNED ~

You feel as if you are having a conversation, partly with the outside world, partly with your inner baby-world. This may make you appear rather vague, even forgetful, at times. Some women worry that their brain is going soft. It isn't. It is just that often you are preoccupied with the other person inside you.

~ DREAMING MORE VIVIDLY ~

Your dreams may be hectic and technicolored, packed with images of water, death, or baby animals. Sometimes they turn into nightmares.

If you already have a child, you may dream of something terrible happening to him or her. Dreams like this occur because you are afraid that you do not have enough love to give to both your older child and the new baby when it arrives.

~ COMMITMENT AND APPREHENSION ~

You feel committed to becoming a mother. This may inspire you to read and find out all you can about birth and babies, get ready for the birth well in advance, and make things for the baby.

You may have a sense of starting out on an adventure. It is exciting, but you are uncertain about what will happen, both at the birth and afterwards.

~ CREATIVITY AND STRENGTH ~

A surge of energy as you approach the birth marks the close of one chapter in your life and the start of a new one. You may tackle work energetically, complete a task with a flourish, or set out on a new creative activity. You may find that your "nesting" instinct becomes stronger, too.

Can't Sleep?

• Your feelings may be so turbulent that you lie awake in the dark. Try these remedies:
• A warm bath to help you unwind. Add a few drops of lavender oil to the water.
• A milk drink or a cup of safe herb tea at bed-time. Be careful not to drink so much that you have to wake up in order to empty your bladder.
• Slow, full breathing. Practice during the peace of the night.

Everything's gone perfectly so far. The doctor says I'm disgustingly healthy. But as I get nearer to the birth I'm beginning to feel that maybe I've been over-confident. It's a kind of stage fright. Actors say that if you feel like that beforehand, you'll be all right on the night!"

"The only thing that's upsetting me is that I'm having a hassle trying to keep control of the birth, especially about getting a home birth. Otherwise I feel great!"

"I want to tell everyone I'm pregnant, I feel so good."

"It sounds disloyal, but I'm determined not to get like my mother. She devoted her whole life to her husband and children. I want to keep some space for myself – me, not just Moshe's wife and the baby's mother."

"I felt exhausted in the first months and thought it would be like that the whole time. Now I feel marvelous. I want to do things! I feel full of energy."

"My last pregnancy was pretty awful, not because I was sick or anything, but because visits to the hospital took forever and made me feel worried and miserable, lacking in confidence, and scared of what they were going to do to me. Having my midwife as a friend has changed this pregnancy. She spends time talking about my feelings, and has gotten to know us as a family. She's warm and caring and calm, so I'm feeling much more positive about myself.

YOUR EMOTIONS NOW

Q What special feelings do you have at this stage of your pregnancy? Describe them here.

_____

_____

_____

_____

_____

_____

_____

_____

_____

_____

_____

_____

_____

_____

_____

_____

_____

_____

_____

TODAY'S DATE _____

THINKING ABOUT LABOR

No one really knows what starts off labor. It may be simply that the uterus cannot grow any more. Natural hormones produced by the placenta, the baby, or both, may play a part, making your finely-tuned body – which for months has nurtured your baby – ready to work to give birth. Labor is an individual experience. Although you will hear about the experiences of other women, your own may be completely different.

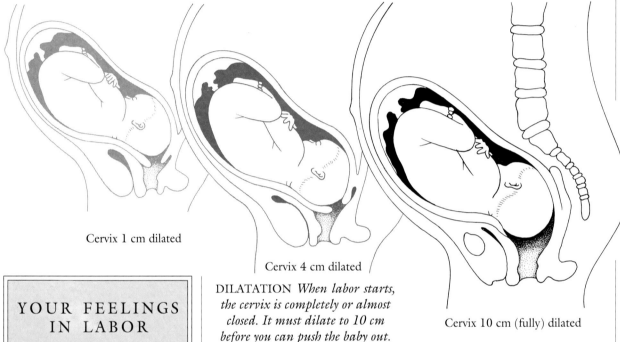

Cervix 1 cm dilated

Cervix 4 cm dilated

DILATATION *When labor starts, the cervix is completely or almost closed. It must dilate to 10 cm before you can push the baby out.*

Cervix 10 cm (fully) dilated

YOUR FEELINGS IN LABOR

When labor starts you may feel very excited. This is it! At about half dilatation you get more serious and focus inward. Between eight and ten centimeters you have to concentrate just to keep going, and may get cranky and irritable. As you start pushing you feel fresh excitement and a flood of energy. Then, with the birth of your baby, there is a rush of emotion: astonishment, relief, thanksgiving, wonder, and triumph.

~ PRE-LABOR CONTRACTIONS ~

The Braxton-Hicks contractions, with which you may be already familiar, are the earliest kind of contraction you may feel. As labor approaches these begin to soften and efface (shorten) your cervix. This is the time to practice relaxation, and to sleep as much as you can.

~ HOW CONTRACTIONS WORK IN LABOR ~

Imagine your uterus as an inflated balloon. If you push down on the top while pulling up the sides with your hands, the bottom stretches up to you. This is what happens with the uterus. Muscles at the top contract, pulling up the lower part so that the cervix opens. The regular strong contractions that you feel when labor has really started open your cervix. They get stronger and closer together, and then – when they are coming about every two minutes – press the baby out through your cervix and vagina.

~ PROS AND CONS OF PAIN-RELIEVING DRUGS ~

You are probably thinking already about whether you will want drugs for relieving pain and, if so, which ones are best.

Demerol, usually given as an injection, takes the edge off pain, but may make you feel drowsy and unable to concentrate. Nausea and vomiting are common, too. The baby sometimes needs help to breathe and may be sleepy and reluctant to suck in the first few days. Phenothiazine (Phenergan) may be added to Demerol to decrease nausea and boost the pain-killing effect, but may disturb the fetal heart-rate.

Epidurals and spinals need to be given by a skilled anesthetist. They anesthetize you from the waist down, although pain may persist in areas that should have been numbed. Occasionally blood pressure drops suddenly, which may make you feel sick and dizzy. The risk of forceps delivery (*see* page 110) is increased.

A pudendal block is an injection of local anesthetic deep inside your vagina. It is given with forceps deliveries when a woman has not already had an epidural, so that she does not feel the birth. Local anesthetic is also used before an episiotomy (*see* page 110), and to repair a tear, but takes a few minutes to work.

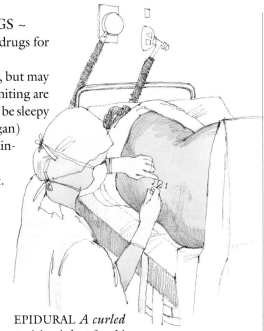

EPIDURAL *A curled position is best for this.*

> *I kept getting Braxton-Hicks contractions. Some were quite painful, so I thought this was it. I phoned the hospital and as we discussed them, I realized that these were pre-labor contractions because they came in clusters, and there wouldn't be any for 20 minutes or so. The midwife said I'd know when I was in labor, since the contractions would get stronger, longer, and closer together.*

> "*My sister says her contractions started like period pains, and later were like a wide elastic band tightening around the bottom of her abdomen. Karen's were all in her back, and Liz had pain down her thighs, too. Nicky said each contraction was like a huge balloon being blown up inside her. When I practice my relaxation and breathing, I imagine all those, so I'm ready for anything!*"

LOOKING AHEAD

Q How are you preparing for the birth of your baby?

_____

_____

_____

_____

Q How do you feel about using drugs to relieve pain in labor?

_____

_____

_____

TODAY'S DATE _____

ENJOYING RELAXATION

WHENEVER YOU CAN, make spaces in your life that are just for you. Use this time for relaxation. It feels good for both body and mind. You conserve energy. Previously scattered thoughts come together. You can focus your imagination on the baby inside you and on how the power of your uterus will open up your body to give birth, so that at last you will be able to see your baby and hold her in your arms.

When I started practicing relaxation, I realized how tense I was. If there were hassles at work, my shoulders tightened, my jaw clenched. Now I drop my shoulders and loosen my jaw.

DEEP RELAXATION *Learning to relax brings a sense of well-being, and you become aware of the baby's unfolding life within you.*

~ RELAXING FOR CHILDBIRTH ~

When you relax in childbirth, and work with your body instead of fighting it, you feel less pain than if you are tense. Your cervix opens more smoothly and your uterus can work better, and because you are not wasting energy you feel less tired when the baby is born. Learning how to relax for childbirth is like learning any other skill. Although you may start off not doing it well, you can become good at it with regular practice. Discovering that you are able to relax will increase your self-confidence.

~ RELEASING TENSION ~

This easy exercise will help you get to know how your body feels when it is relaxed. Sit or lie, propped up with plenty of pillows, in any position in which it feels comfortable to sleep. The small of your back and your neck should be supported, your shoulders rounded, and your head dropped slightly forward like a heavy flower on its stem.

Then pull your shoulders down, feeling the pull at the back of your neck, and allow them to settle back easily into position. Let your neck muscles be loose, your jaw dropped, and just listen to the sound of your breathing.

As you continue breathing slowly and fully, think over all the different parts of your body and let any tension flow out of them: your hands, feet, thighs, bottom, abdomen, arms, the muscles around your eyes and mouth – every single part of you. Enjoy the feeling of peace when you have released all muscular tension.

TOUCH AND MASSAGE

You may enjoy an abdominal or lower back massage with a little oil while you visualize your baby inside you. You can add a few drops of essential oil to a light vegetable oil (soy or almond) for a delicious scented massage. Geranium or rose are especially pleasant.

The massage can be a deeply sensual experience, and help you store energy and confidence for all that lies ahead.

As you relax, tension flows out from the center of the body towards the periphery – muscles near the surface of the skin – and disappears. The massaging hands can help this by emphasizing movements of stroking down and outwards, and making upward or inward strokes light.

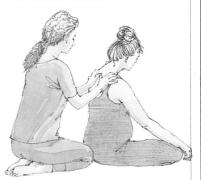

SHOULDER MASSAGE
Your helper massages with both thumbs in the spaces at either side of the top of your spine.

Gentle abdominal massage will help you relax and get in touch with the baby, too. Think of your baby responding to the touch. From now on, you may notice that the baby seems to move and kick as if being stroked and played with. Sometimes it seems as though the baby is even playing with the massaging hands. For a father, his first delighted meeting with the baby may be through touch like this.

How to Massage

- Always massage with relaxed arms and hands.
- Massage slowly, molding your hands to the shape of the body.
- Use firm pressure in the small of the back, light pressure on the abdomen.
- When using firm touch, don't tighten the muscles in your arms, but allow the weight of your upper back to flow through your relaxed arms down into the part of the body you are massaging.

ARM MASSAGE
Supporting your arm at the wrist, your helper massages the muscle of your inside upper arm slowly and firmly.

I have a bath, then lie on a rug on the floor and Chris massages me gently all over with a special oil."

"It's time together for us and the baby. We're getting to know our baby through touch."

"Learning to relax, and having these regular, luxurious massages, has helped me feel a calmer person, more centered.

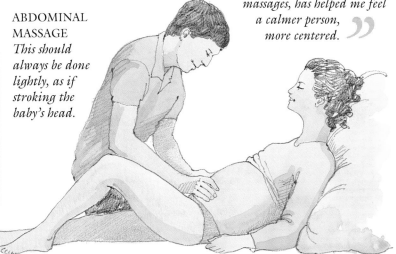

ABDOMINAL MASSAGE
This should always be done lightly, as if stroking the baby's head.

Weeks 25 *to* 28

B Y 28 WEEKS leg veins may be more marked. Varicose veins may appear. This is partly hereditary, partly due to pregnancy hormones softening valves in the veins. It can't be prevented, but you can avoid standing around, and lie with legs raised above your pelvis so that blood-flow back to your heart is easier. The softening and stretching of pelvic ligaments may result in a backache. Keep your spine straight, and think of your head balancing like a ball on top of your neck vertebrae.

Body Facts

• There may be red streaks where your skin has stretched, especially on your abdomen, bottom, and breasts.
• Half of all pregnant women get heartburn at this stage. It feels like fire in your throat, and is caused by progesterone softening a valve in your digestive tract, so that acid rises from your stomach. Have small meals, and avoid bending and lying flat on your back.

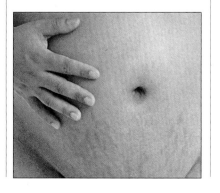

" I feel I've turned into a squashy, bulging earth mother figure."

"I've never felt so positive about my body, so fulfilled."

STRETCH MARKS
These fade and turn silver after the birth.

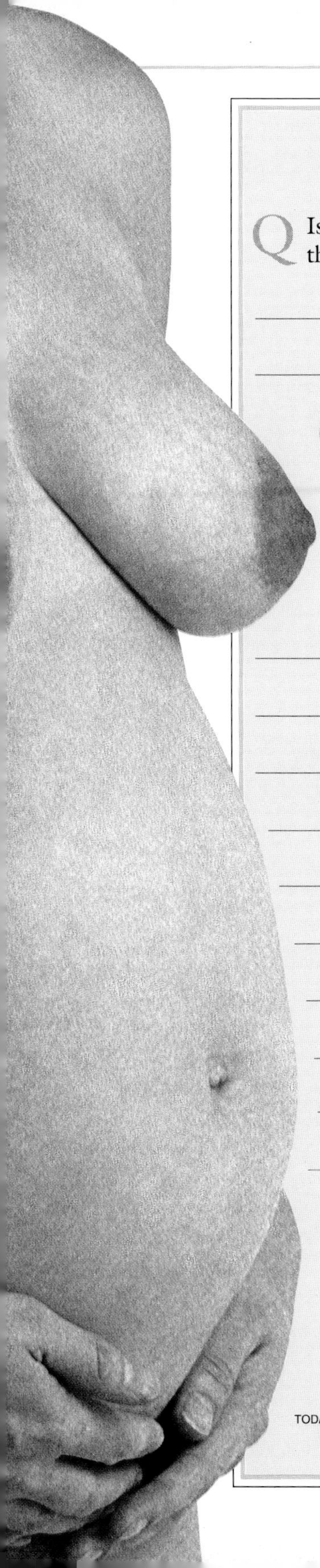

LOOKING BACK

Q Is this stage of pregnancy much as you thought it would be?

_____

_____

Q Has anything occurred that is different from what you expected, or hoped for?

_____

_____

_____

_____

_____

_____

_____

_____

_____

_____

_____

TODAY'S DATE _____

Week 25   MONTH / DAY / YEAR

S
M
T
W
T
F
S

Week 26   MONTH / DAY / YEAR

S
M
T
W
T
F
S

Week 27   MONTH / DAY / YEAR

S
M
T
W
T
F
S

Week 28   MONTH / DAY / YEAR

S
M
T
W
T
F
S

HOW YOUR BABY IS GROWING

BY 28 WEEKS the baby is able to hear much more. In early pregnancy, the nerve endings that enable sound to be heard were not yet connected, so she experienced sound as strong vibration, as if from the twanging strings of a cello or guitar.

People used to think that it was quiet inside the uterus. Now it is known that it is a noisy place, like a busy railway station, a factory, or the engine room of a ship. There are the gurglings and rumble of your digestive system, and the pumping sounds that come from your beating heart and your lungs as they expand and contract. If you walk around or have a party, it's even noisier. Throughout pregnancy the uterus trembles with vibrations, too.

When you speak, your voice goes down into your body as well as out. The baby's heart beats faster when you speak, too. The baby gets accustomed to the sound of your voice and can recognize it immediately after birth. Even so, your voice may be muffled because vernix, a protective thick cream which often still clings to the baby's body at birth, plugs the ears.

Fine, downy hair covers her body. It is patterned like ripples left by waves on the sand.

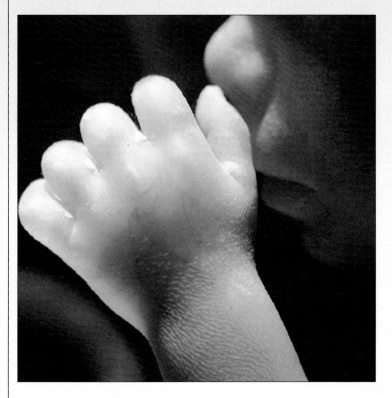

PARCHMENT-LIKE SKIN
Tiny veins are visible through the baby's translucent skin.

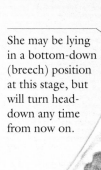

She may be lying in a bottom-down (breech) position at this stage, but will turn head-down any time from now on.

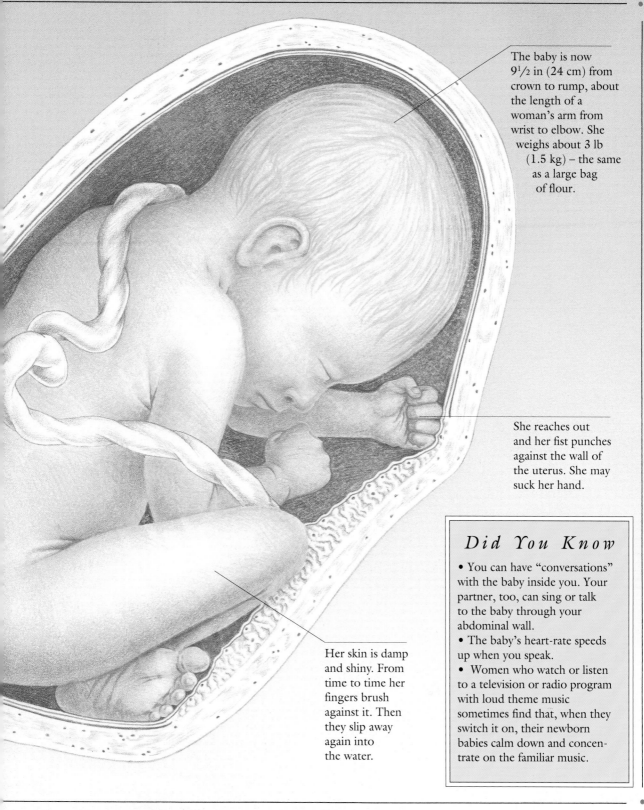

The baby is now 9¹/₂ in (24 cm) from crown to rump, about the length of a woman's arm from wrist to elbow. She weighs about 3 lb (1.5 kg) – the same as a large bag of flour.

She reaches out and her fist punches against the wall of the uterus. She may suck her hand.

Her skin is damp and shiny. From time to time her fingers brush against it. Then they slip away again into the water.

Did You Know

• You can have "conversations" with the baby inside you. Your partner, too, can sing or talk to the baby through your abdominal wall.

• The baby's heart-rate speeds up when you speak.

• Women who watch or listen to a television or radio program with loud theme music sometimes find that, when they switch it on, their newborn babies calm down and concentrate on the familiar music.

EMOTIONAL CHALLENGES

Y OU MAY FEEL VERY CALM about the approaching birth. Yet most women have times when they feel like they are on the edge of a mountain, with uncharted space in front of them. It is exciting and scary. You ask yourself: *Will I be able to stand the pain? What will "they" do to me? Will the baby be all right? Can I be a good mother?* It is good to talk about your feelings with other pregnant women and couples, which is one reason why classes that encourage open and free discussion are helpful. Being aware of challenges enables you to develop strategies to meet them.

Why do you Feel Like This?

• Anxiety about the birth is a stimulus to negotiate the kind of care you want in a confident, assertive way, and to learn all you can and how to handle pain positively.
• Increased sensitivity, and the ease with which tears flow, are signs that you are in the heightened emotional state that makes a mother especially responsive to a newborn baby.
• All the strong emotions you feel now can help you prepare for the changes ahead.

~ WILL I BE ABLE TO STAND THE PAIN? ~

You may worry that you have a low pain threshold, or that you have never had to cope with pain before. If your mother had a bad time in childbirth, perhaps you are anxious that it will be the same for you. This fear does not need to be wasted. You can use it constructively to learn how to relax and breathe, and work in harmony with the power of your uterus.

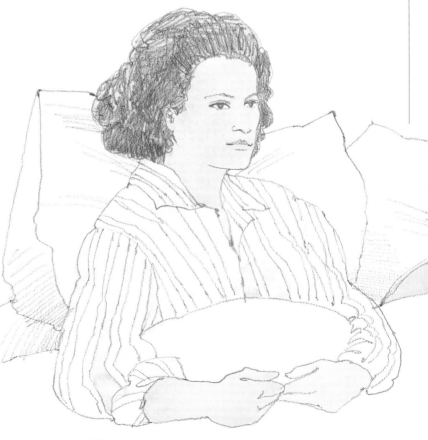

" *Tim and I are very much in love. We're thrilled about the baby, but we don't want our relationship to change. I've seen so many couples drift apart when children come and I don't want that to happen. There are nagging thoughts in the back of my mind: Will he still love me? and Am I going to feel torn between him and the baby's needs?*"

"*I lie in the dark and worry that the baby might be abnormal. I feel that if I talk about it, it will somehow make it more likely to happen.*"

~ WHAT WILL "THEY" DO TO ME? ~

If you don't know who will be caring for you during childbirth, you may be concerned that professionals will make decisions for you, and that you will be "processed" through labor as if on a conveyor belt.

Ask other women about their experiences and contact childbirth organizations and women's groups to learn how to get the kind of care and birth place you want. Some useful addresses are listed on page 127.

~ WILL THE BABY BE ALL RIGHT? ~

It may seem impossible that your body can produce a perfect baby, especially if you are not confident of your own worth, and feel you can't live up to standards set by other people. Awareness of dangers in our polluted world may make you worry that something you ate, breathed, or did, has harmed your baby. These anxieties express your feelings of responsibility for your baby. In fact, most babies are miraculously perfect.

~ CAN I BE A GOOD MOTHER? ~

With the first baby, you may doubt if you have any maternal instincts. You may not enjoy other people's children much. If yours was a small family, you probably never had babies around as you were growing up, so you could not become confident in handling them. Mothering is learned behavior. You will need your baby close to you after the birth, and to have plenty of time to watch and interact with this little person. Then your baby will soon *show* you how to be a good mother.

After I had George I suffered from depression, and felt very detached from the baby for the first six months. I feel like I failed him. I'm afraid this could happen again. It's the reason I'm having a home birth, but I'm still anxious.

MOTHERING SKILLS
Knowing how to be a mother comes from contact with children, and from developing confidence in caring for them.

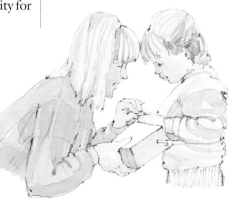

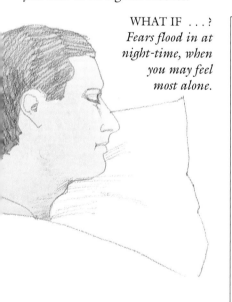

WHAT IF . . .?
Fears flood in at night-time, when you may feel most alone.

SHARING YOUR FEARS

Q Do you have any fears or worries that you want to talk about with someone close to you, or in classes?

_____

_____

_____

_____

_____

TODAY'S DATE _____

BIRTH PLANS

A BIRTH PLAN IS A LIST you make of things that are important to you about the birth of your baby and the time afterwards. It is best to base it on discussion with those caring for you, rather than merely to hand it to them. It shouldn't be like an ultimatum or a lengthy shopping list. One copy is inserted in your records. You keep some others with the things you have ready for the birth and hand one to each person who cares for you during labor. Where there is continuity of care and you get to know a midwife or doctor in pregnancy, and trust and like each other, a Birth Plan may be unnecessary. But if you are going to meet people when you are in labor whom you have not met before, a Birth Plan will help them know your wishes.

Procedures that may be used in Labor

- Continuous electronic fetal monitoring.

- Amniotomy (having your waters broken).

- Oxytocin stimulation to stimulate (speed up) labor.

- An intravenous drip to feed glucose or drugs into your bloodstream.

- Drugs for pain relief (Demerol, Vistaril, epidural).

- Episiotomy (being cut).

- Planned Cesarean section (with either general anesthesia or an epidural).

- Forceps or vacuum extraction.

FIND OUT ALL YOU CAN
Discuss the things that matter most to you with the midwife or doctor. Ask what their experience is of different procedures, why they consider some routines useful, and why they have, perhaps, abandoned others that were once the rule. Then record your wishes in a Birth Plan.

~ THINKING ABOUT YOUR OWN PLAN ~

Some issues you may want to include are: the people you would like with you during labor; what is most important to you about the conduct of your labor; your thoughts about procedures that may be used in labor; what you would like to have in the birth room; things you would like to be able to do (for example, be free to move around); how much private time you would like with your baby; and how you want to feed her.

Look back at what you wrote in Your Choices on pages 16–17. Then use the questions on pages 82–83 to make notes for composing your own plan. Write it on a separate sheet of paper, and make as many copies as you need.

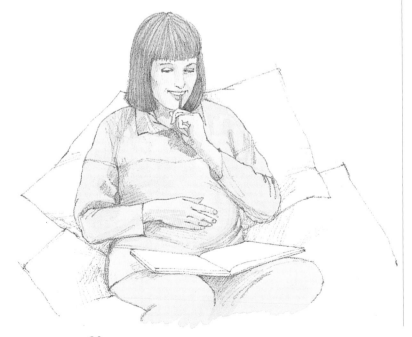

80

~ MAKING CONTINGENCY PLANS ~

When you plan a picnic you make alternative arrangements in case it rains heavily. It is the same when you are thinking ahead to labor. If a birth is complicated, or longer or more painful or difficult than expected, or if the baby needs to go to the special care nursery, it is useful to have ideas about what you would want in these different circumstances. Being aware of these possibilities does not make them more likely to happen, but does help you cope more effectively if labor brings surprises.

Unless there is a good chance that you will need a Cesarean, or that the baby will require special care, you do not need to have a written account of your wishes about these in your records. But make sure that your birth partner knows what you want, and has the confidence to express your preferences in case it is difficult for you to do so at the time.

They consulted my Birth Plan, discussed everything with me, and I felt they were on my side."

"The doctor raised her eyebrows when she saw my Birth Plan and said, 'You've been reading books!' I laughed and said, 'Don't you?' She replied, 'It's my job.' 'Well,' I said, 'having a baby is mine at the moment – and I want to do it as well as I can.'

TWO WOMEN'S BIRTH PLANS

BIRTH CHOICES *These two sample Plans show how you can help your caregivers know your wishes.*

Thank you for the information you have provided in the prenatal clinic and at the classes at Central Hospital. I have found this very helpful, and after discussion with the midwives I would like to record my wishes about the birth, as they have suggested. They are:

That the support person I've chosen to be with me, my sister, will be with me at all times, including if I need an assisted delivery. She has been to some of the classes with me, and has three children herself.

I would like to be able to go into labor spontaneously and not be induced, because that experience was very unpleasant last time.

I understand that it is routine practice to use the external electronic monitor for 20 minutes or so on admission, and I am happy for that to be done, but do not want scalp electrodes on the baby's head.

If I need drugs for pain relief, I prefer an epidural to Demerol, with as low an anesthetic dose as possible, so that I still have feeling in my legs and am aware of contractions. I'd like to let it wear off for the second stage, since I hope to be able to push the baby out myself.

If everything goes well, on the other hand, and I don't need pain relief, I would like to walk around and to give birth standing up.

I'm grateful for all the help and encouragement you can give me.

Signed: Lisa Robinson

I'm looking forward to coming into St Stephen's to have my baby. I have thought carefully about what I would like during childbirth and have had help in thinking things through from my doctor. We have agreed that:

My partner, Douglas, and a woman friend of mine, Katy, who has attended childbirth classes with me will be my companions during labor.

I will ask for pain-killing drugs if I feel I need them, but prefer them not to be offered to me otherwise.

I would like to move around and have a bean-bag and mat from the physiotherapy department on the floor for both the first and second stages of labor if everything is proceeding normally.

With this in mind, I do not want to have an internal fetal monitor or anything which involves strapping me down.

I hope to manage without an episiotomy and to give birth with an intact perineum if possible, and welcome help to achieve this.

If the baby is in good condition at birth, the airways will not be sucked out.

Since I am going to breastfeed, I do not want the baby to be given water or formula.

I will have 24 hour rooming-in and would like to do everything for the baby myself.

I appreciate all the help and encouragement you can give me to achieve the kind of birth for which I am hoping.

Signed: Janet Morley

MAKING YOUR BIRTH PLAN

Q Who would you like with you at the birth?

_____

Q What is most important to you about your labor?

_____

_____

_____

Q Do you want to be kept fully informed and share in any discussions and decisions made?

_____

Q Are there any things you would like to have in the birth room?

_____

_____

_____

EXTERNAL FETAL HEART MONITOR
This also records contractions at the same time.

Q Do you have any special requests of those caring for you?

_____

_____

_____

Q What are your thoughts about procedures that may be used during labor?

_____

_____

_____

_____

Q Do you have any special requests about the delivery?

_____

_____

_____

Q Is there anything that it is important for you to be able to do during labor?

_____

_____

_____

Q What other things are important to you about the birth itself?

_____

_____

_____

Q Do you want the third stage of labor to be speeded up medically, or would you prefer to deliver the afterbirth naturally?

_____

SQUATTING BAR This gives you good support while you squat or kneel to push.

Q Do you have any special wishes about the hour immediately after birth?

_____

_____

_____

Q Do you want to be awakened at night to feed your baby?

_____

Q Do you have any special requests about feeding your baby?

_____

_____

Q In the hours and days after, how much time would you like with your baby?

_____

_____

Q What other things are important to you about the time after the birth?

_____

_____

Q Would you like your baby in bed with you, beside your bed, or in the nursery?

_____

_____

_____

Q How do you want to feed your baby?

_____

_____

TODAY'S DATE _____

Weeks 29 *to* 32

YOUR HEART IS NOW WORKING about 25% harder than before pregnancy, and blood volume is up by almost 3 quarts (2.5 liters). Because there is added pressure on blood vessels in the lower half of the body, some women have hemorrhoids, or varicose veins in the legs or vulva. Because your stomach empties more slowly, a heavy meal leaves you feeling bloated. You may notice increased vaginal secretions. Pelvic joints are softening and stretching ready for the birth, so you are comfortable only in low-heeled shoes. Your uterus is tightening regularly in readiness for the birth, too, sometimes so hard that you catch your breath. These very firm squeezes of your abdomen are called "Braxton-Hicks contractions".

Body Facts

- You can help the softening of the tissues of your vagina, labia and perineum, and make them more flexible, by massaging them daily with wheatgerm oil.
- Ligaments attached to your pelvis loosen with the action of pregnancy hormones, so that a large baby can pass through a relatively small pelvis.
- Stretching of ligaments can often result in a backache. An all-fours position usually relieves it.
- You can rehearse breathing and relaxation with Braxton-Hicks contractions once they are long and strong.

I was beginning to worry how the family would cope while I was in the hospital. So we had some good cooking sessions, making double quantities of everything and putting half in the freezer just in case the baby came early.

"I showed John how to feel the baby. Now we lie in bed and cuddle and he can feel the baby's firm rounded back and knobby feet.

HELPING YOUR BODY

Q What things are you doing to help yourself be physically comfortable?

_____

_____

_____

_____

_____

_____

_____

_____

Q How are you preparing your body for the birth?

_____

_____

_____

_____

_____

_____

_____

_____

_____

TODAY'S DATE _____

Week 29 MONTH / DAY / YEAR

S
M
T
W
T
F
S

Week 30 MONTH / DAY / YEAR

S
M
T
W
T
F
S

Week 31 MONTH / DAY / YEAR

S
M
T
W
T
F
S

Week 32 MONTH / DAY / YEAR

S
M
T
W
T
F
S

HOW YOUR BABY IS GROWING

BY 32 WEEKS most babies have turned head-down in the uterus. They do this after about 28 weeks, and stay that way until birth. Others don't, and stay head-up in the uterus for a little longer. A minority of babies remain fixed like this so that they are born bottom-first. A head-down position is called "vertex" or "cephalic", and a bottom-down position is called "breech". The illustration on pages 76–77 shows a baby lying in a breech position. Other vertex and breech positions are illustrated on pages 98–99.

A small baby who has a good deal of space in the uterus may still be changing from breech to vertex and back for a few more weeks. Sometimes when a baby does not fix head-down, it is a sign that you are not as advanced in pregnancy as you first thought.

You will know when your baby is lying head-down because you feel feet kicking against your ribs instead of the hard ball of the baby's head. Once he has settled head-down, the baby may bounce his head against your springy pelvic floor muscles, at first gently, and then – as he drops lower into your pelvis – more and more vigorously.

Did You Know

• If your baby is breech, your doctor may be able to turn it. Or you can try tipping the baby out of your pelvis by getting into a head-down position, which may encourage it to somersault.
• The easiest way is to lie on your front with your hips raised on a sofa, and your head and shoulders on the floor. You'll need to lie like this for 20 minutes two or three times a day, so have some music on, or magazines to flip through, or you may get bored.

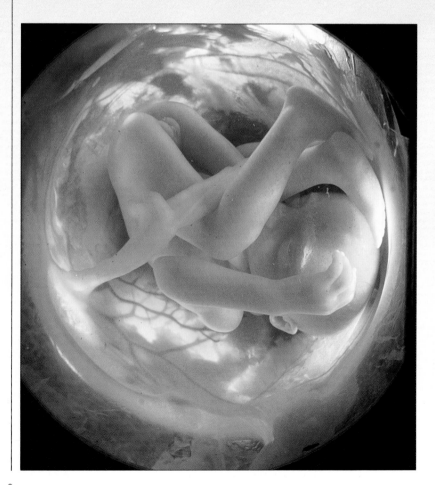

GETTING TO KNOW YOUR BABY *As pregnancy advances, you become more aware of different parts of the baby: his kicking feet, round head, strong, curved back, and stubby bottom.*

The baby's head bounces against the cervix. It feels round like a ball.

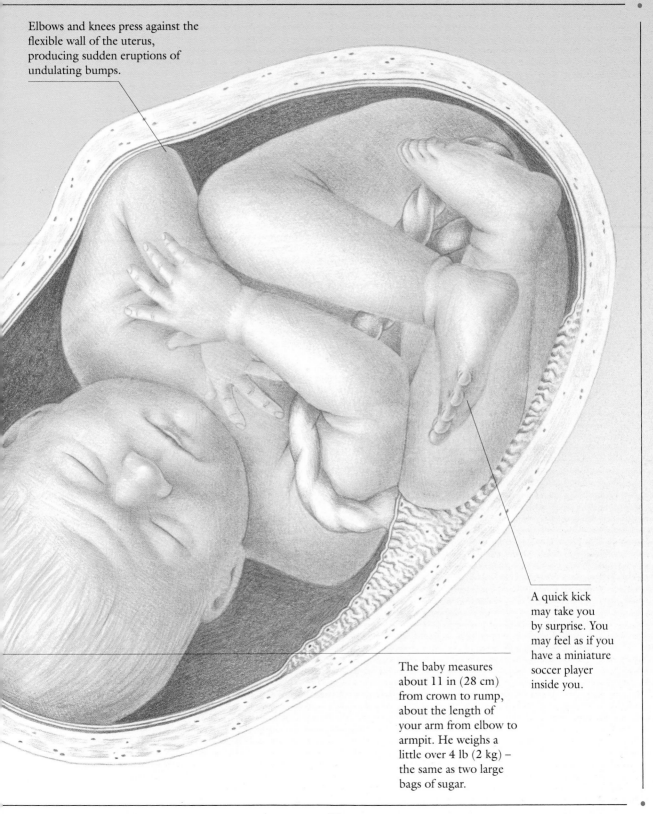

Elbows and knees press against the flexible wall of the uterus, producing sudden eruptions of undulating bumps.

A quick kick may take you by surprise. You may feel as if you have a miniature soccer player inside you.

The baby measures about 11 in (28 cm) from crown to rump, about the length of your arm from elbow to armpit. He weighs a little over 4 lb (2 kg) – the same as two large bags of sugar.

BREATHING RHYTHMS

BEING AWARE OF YOUR BREATHING helps you relax. In labor it enables you to co-ordinate with the contractions of your uterus, as if you were swimming over large, swelling waves. Breathing for childbirth isn't a matter of exercise, but of harmonizing breathing with relaxation and opening. Because breathing and relaxation are interdependent, they are best practiced together.

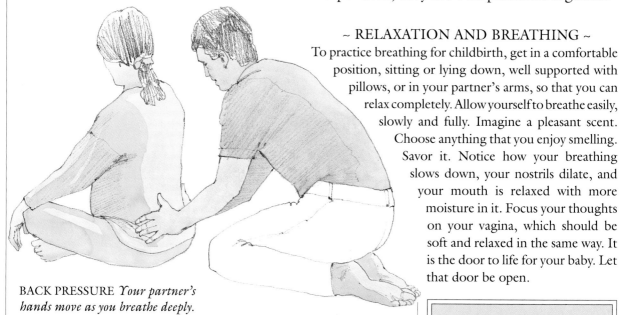

~ RELAXATION AND BREATHING ~

To practice breathing for childbirth, get in a comfortable position, sitting or lying down, well supported with pillows, or in your partner's arms, so that you can relax completely. Allow yourself to breathe easily, slowly and fully. Imagine a pleasant scent. Choose anything that you enjoy smelling. Savor it. Notice how your breathing slows down, your nostrils dilate, and your mouth is relaxed with more moisture in it. Focus your thoughts on your vagina, which should be soft and relaxed in the same way. It is the door to life for your baby. Let that door be open.

BACK PRESSURE *Your partner's hands move as you breathe deeply.*

~ BREATHING IN THE FIRST STAGE OF LABOR ~

Listen to the sound of your breathing, like waves rolling on the seashore. Relax more with each breath out. Let each breath in help you focus your thoughts deep in your body. As you breathe out, visualize your cervix softening, opening and stretching wide so that your baby can press through. These mental images can help you through the first stage of labor.

~ THE FINAL OPENING OF THE CERVIX ~

Imagine that you are having a strong contraction now. Remain relaxed while your breathing gets lighter and quicker. Then, as the contraction fades, breathe slowly and fully, right down to where your baby is waiting to be born. In the interval between contractions, relax completely.

Many women find that their breathing gets faster at the height of strong contractions at the end of the first stage. If this is how it is for you, let your breathing be quick but also light. Greet each contraction with slow, full breathing, keep any rapid breathing as light as a whisper, and always return to slow, full breathing as the contraction eases.

Breathing for Birth

- If your breathing becomes faster as contractions get stronger, make sure it is lighter. Let it "dance".
- Give a long, slow breath out – the welcoming breath – with the start of each contraction.
- Give a long, slow breath out as each contraction disappears.
- If you feel you are running out of breath, drop your shoulders and give a few long breaths out and in to regain the rhythm.
- You may prefer to sing, chant, roar, or shout. All these work well, especially if the sounds are deep rather than shrill.

> *I couldn't relax before I was pregnant and thought lying around was a waste of time. Now I enjoy it. Sometimes I sing and talk to the baby, too. I feel that rather than doing special breathing in labor, it will come naturally for me to sing and moan, and my midwife says that's fine."*

> *"John gives a wonderful foot massage. I tend to over-breathe when I get anxious. But when he massages my feet, I breathe more gently and evenly.*

~ BREATHING FOR PUSHING ~

Now take a full breath and hold it for four or five seconds and see if you can stay relaxed. You will feel pressure in your body, but keep your shoulders spaced wide and loose, lips apart and jaw dropped, legs and arms relaxed. Then breathe out. Breathe easily for a while. Then repeat the held breath, staying soft and loose, and imagining the tissues of your vagina spreading out and opening as the baby's head presses through.

~ HOW EASY BREATHING HELPS YOUR BABY ~

A good supply of oxygen is vital for your baby's well-being. It is carried in blood flowing through the placenta into the umbilical cord. If you get very tense, blood surges to your brain, heart, and arm and leg muscles, and is reduced in the placenta. So the baby may have less oxygen for a while. For some babies, this seems to set up a pattern that leads them to have disturbed sleep rhythms after they are born, and be irritable and hard to comfort. Learning how to relax and manage stress is one way of soothing your baby while she is still inside your uterus.

BREATHING THE BABY OUT

Gasping and heavy panting, caused by pain and panic, flushes carbon dioxide out of the bloodstream and disturbs the blood's acid balance. A woman over-breathing like this becomes dizzy, has tingling fingers, numb lips, and may even black out. Rhythmic easy breathing is best.

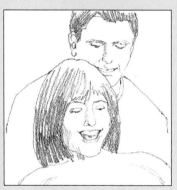

As the head appears, drop your jaw and breathe your baby out.

If you want to breathe quickly as you approach full dilatation, make this rapid breathing as light as you can. When you are pushing, hold your breath only for as long as you want. As the head starts to slide out, instead of pushing, drop your jaw and *breathe* your baby out.

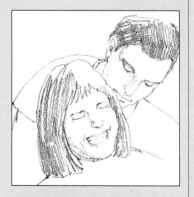

Hold your breath no longer than six seconds for each push.

> *My legs got tense and I started to hyperventilate. John stroked firmly and slowly down my inside legs, up lightly, and then down again."*

> *"I knelt up, leaning over, every time a contraction came. Each one felt like going up to the top of a mountain, and my breathing got shallower and faster. José began giving firm pressure in the small of my back. It made an unbelievable difference to the discomfort I felt with each contraction! And it was soothing in between because I was experiencing a lot of low back pain all the time."*

> *"It was difficult to go on breathing through those contractions, because at their height they took my breath away. Every time I lost the rhythm I sought Amy's eyes and she breathed with me, and I got back into it again.*

THE BABY'S MOVEMENTS

THE BABY ROLLS, TUMBLES, kicks, bounces, and even hiccups inside you. Movements that you felt as mere flutterings in earlier weeks now become thumps and bumps. The baby pushes a foot against the springy wall of your uterus. She turns over from one side to the other and somersaults. She loses her thumb and turns her head rapidly from side to side in a reflex movement to find something to suck. Sometimes a baby kicks so much that you feel sore under your ribs.

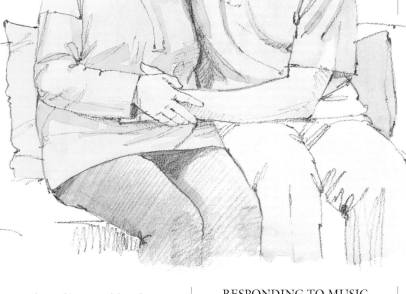

~ BEING AWARE OF YOUR BABY ~

Many babies become active and seem to bounce around when their mothers lie down for a rest, soak in a bath, or go to bed at night. Evening is also a time when babies often kick, turn and thump more than earlier in the day. If your baby is like this while inside you, it may come as no surprise that, a few weeks after birth, your baby has a wakeful spell in the evenings, when you would like to be able to sit down and take a break.

There are times when the baby is less active. If the weather is hot, your baby may seem drowsy, and you may notice that she is particularly quiet after you have eaten a heavy meal. Babies move less, too, when their mothers drink a lot of alcohol or smoke.

~ STRONG EMOTIONS ~

You may have realized that your baby responds to your strong emotions, too. If you are frightened, or get very upset or excited about something, for example, stress hormones are released in your bloodstream, and can pass through the placenta into the baby. They stimulate an increased heart-rate and movements in the baby. Women who are under severe emotional stress sometimes have jumpy babies. But strong emotions are part of being human. If you notice that the baby is very active when you are angry or stressed, try to give yourself some time to relax and breathe slowly, so that you and your baby can quiet down. You can comfort and communicate love to your baby in this way while she is still inside you. When it's difficult to go and rest, simply relax where you are, swaying gently.

RESPONDING TO MUSIC
Just when you want to share the thrill of the leaping life you feel inside you, the movements may stop. See what happens when you and your partner sing to the baby or play music. Babies may show preferences in music – some respond to a military band, while others like rock music or a violin concerto.

"The baby always shuffles around if I lie on my back and makes me uncomfortable. It doesn't seem to like it, so I have to turn over on to my side. That's more comfortable for me, too, usually."

"There's a kind of rat-a-tat-tat and I'm not sure what it is. It's quite different from the usual lurches, shuffles, and kicks. Almost as if he's knocking to come out."

"The baby's very low now and sometimes it feels as if its hair is tickling inside my vagina. Every so often there's a sharp feeling like a slight electric shock. My childbirth teacher says the baby is probably bouncing its head against my pelvic muscles and getting into a good position for birth."

"My baby is lying with its spine against mine, so I feel most of the kicking at the front. I thought at first it must be twins because there was so much movement, but then my midwife explained that there was a dip, like a saucer, around my own navel, and that was the space between the arms and legs, so the baby is posterior. With the amount of energetic activity I'm feeling, I think the baby will kick itself around by the time I go into labor."

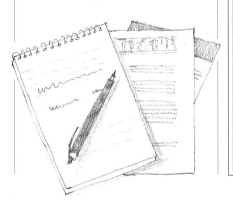

~ REACTING TO SOUND ~

If you go to a concert, or are listening to loud music at home, or if fireworks are being set off, or even if your older children are just having a noisy fight, the baby may respond by leaping around as if excited by the sound. Babies are not completely insulated from the world outside and start being members of the family even before they are born.

~ FEELING MOVEMENTS ~

Your midwife and doctor are interested in your baby's activity and may ask how the movements are at each visit. You often do not notice the baby kicking so much at the end of pregnancy because your growing baby has less space in which to move and because she has become such a part of your life that it would seem unnatural not to feel them. Once the baby is born, you may miss the closeness of these movements and feel lonely without them.

HOW YOUR BABY MOVES

Q At what times of the day or night does your baby seem to move most?

_____

_____

Q How would you describe the different kinds of movement your baby makes?

_____

_____

Q When are your baby's quiet times?

_____

_____

_____

TODAY'S DATE _____

YOUR BLOOD PRESSURE

Blood pressure often rises slightly at the end of pregnancy because of the extra demands made on your metabolism. This does not harm you or the baby. High blood pressure – hypertension – is not a disease, but a sign that some part of the body is not working well. In pregnancy it may mean that the placenta is not functioning as efficiently as it should. Your caregivers will want to see you more often, and may suggest that you get more rest.

~ COPING WITH RAISED BLOOD PRESSURE ~

Blood pressure will usually drop if you can avoid stress. Relax in bed and pamper yourself. Practice relaxation and slow, full breathing. Visualize the baby nestling comfortably inside you. Get someone else to do your shopping, and, if possible, sleep every afternoon in a darkened room. Try taking 1,000 mgs of vitamin C and 400 mgs of vitamin E daily.

~ HYPERTENSION AND PRE-ECLAMPSIA ~

If your blood pressure is high, or if there is a steep rise from early pregnancy, your doctor and midwife will monitor you closely, although you probably feel perfectly well. If a condition called pre-eclampsia develops, where your blood pressure rises further, you have protein in your urine, puffiness under your skin from fluid retention, and a sudden gain in weight, you will be admitted to the hospital to rest, and may be given drugs to reduce your blood pressure. These sometimes have a side-effect of making you feel sedated. Labor may be induced while the baby is still healthy. If pre-eclampsia becomes severe, you may need a Cesarean section (see page 111).

RELAXING BODY AND MIND
Rest can reduce raised blood pressure. Music may help you relax, and sometimes it is easier to release tension if you are doing something with your hands. Or you might imagine a peaceful scene – a forest glade or coral beach – and lying down on soft ferns or white sand while you listen to birds singing, or the rush of waves.

"Doctors think my little girl was stillborn because of severe pre-eclampsia. I was induced and she looked perfect. I just couldn't understand it because I'd felt so well."

"I hate going to the hospital clinic – each time my blood pressure goes up. Everyone tells me to rest more. I'd like to see them try to rest with two children under four."

Pre-eclampsia

You are less likely to develop pre-eclampsia if:

• You already have a baby by the same partner.
• No one in your family has high blood pressure.
• You haven't had high blood pressure in a previous pregnancy.
• You don't get migraines.

PREMATURE BABIES

WITH MODERN TECHNOLOGY and skilled care, babies born as early as 24 weeks survive. But the fight for their lives and health is stressful for everyone. At 24 weeks a baby has a 40-70 percent chance of survival, and by 26 weeks, an 80-90 percent chance. Babies who do well later often have breathing difficulties at first, and take some time to learn how to suck.

~ LOOKING AT A SPECIAL CARE BABY UNIT ~

In an intensive care baby unit, monitors tick, lights flash, occasionally an alarm sounds, and tubes coil around the babies' bodies and into their noses and mouths. What you are seeing are life-support systems designed to take over the functions of the mother's body and placenta.

~ CARING FOR YOUR PREMATURE BABY ~

In many modern units you can ask to have a room nearby and to help care for your baby. The advantage is that you can soothe him after painful treatment, sing to and stroke him, and – when he can be lifted out of the plastic box – cuddle and rock him. Doing this, you can provide the stimulation and comforting that starts off your loving relationship.

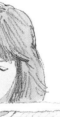

I'M YOUR MOTHER
You can show love even when your baby is in an incubator.

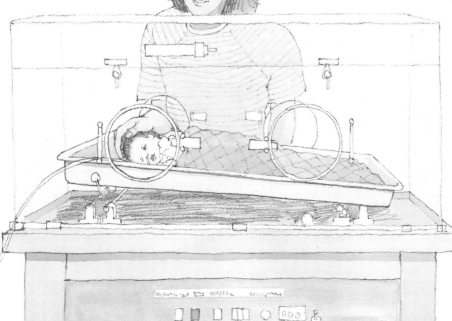

"He looked like a little frog, all wired up on a ventilator. I felt very guilty that I hadn't held on to him safely inside me."

"To be honest, I didn't feel anything except the kind of pity you'd feel for a wounded animal. Her skin was red and shiny, and her eyes were tight shut. She didn't seem human to me."

"The staff in the intensive care unit was wonderful. When she was out of the incubator I tried to do things for her. I was all thumbs. She didn't feel like my baby. It wasn't until we got home that she really belonged to me."

"The nurse said, 'Hold her against your body and talk to her – it helps her grow.' She was so tiny and was being fed through a tube. I held her against my bare skin, let her smell my breast, and she started to lick it as if she was intrigued. My breasts got hot. I felt milk welling up and it started to drip. I knew then that I was going to be able to feed her, that we had a special relationship. It was only five days later that we got breastfeeding going."

Weeks 33 *to* 36

B Y 36 WEEKS you may feel very heavy. While the baby is high, it is difficult to breathe deeply, as its bottom presses against your diaphragm and ribcage. This eases when, any time from now, the baby's head engages in your pelvis. After this, the ball of the head rests against your bladder, so you have to urinate more often. Lying flat on your back you may feel nauseous and dizzy because the heavy uterus presses on a large blood vessel, and slows down the flow of blood back to your heart. It is better to lie on your side or well propped up. Sleep may be interrupted, too. You have short naps rather than a long sleep – good preparation for the time after the baby is born.

Body Facts

• A dark line from your navel down may show where the muscle at the front of your abdomen has stretched. When the muscle "zips" up again after the birth, and your muscles are well toned, this disappears.
• Colostrum – the first kind of milk, specially rich in protein – may leak from your breasts.
• It is normal to retain some fluid under the skin and have slightly swollen ankles, especially in hot weather. If you are getting very puffy, show your doctor or midwife.

Now I'm impatient! Part of me hopes the baby will come early, but I realize that's selfish because his lungs might not be mature enough for him to breathe on his own. I've started a patchwork quilt to see how many squares I can do before the birth.

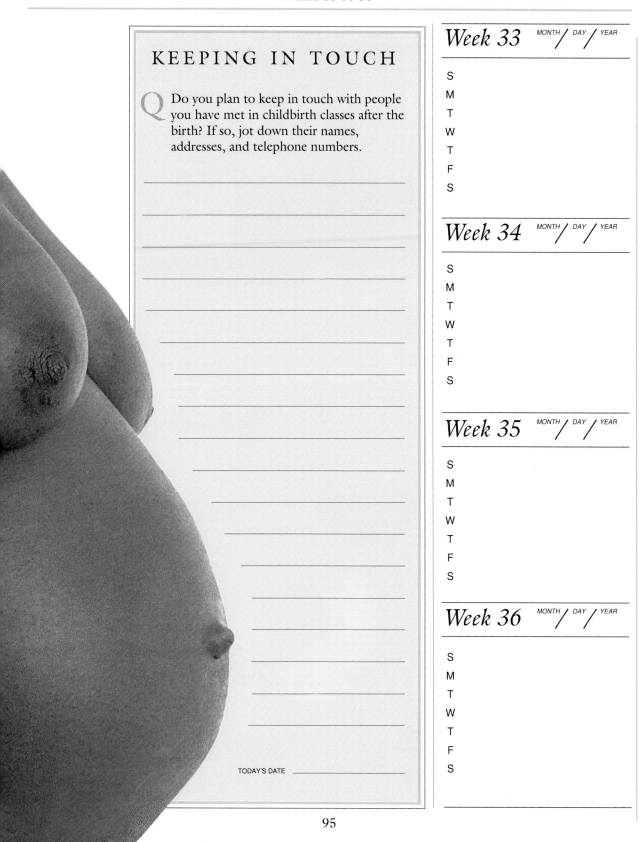

KEEPING IN TOUCH

Q Do you plan to keep in touch with people you have met in childbirth classes after the birth? If so, jot down their names, addresses, and telephone numbers.

_____

_____

_____

_____

_____

_____

_____

_____

_____

_____

_____

_____

_____

_____

_____

_____

TODAY'S DATE _____

Week 33   MONTH / DAY / YEAR

S
M
T
W
T
F
S

Week 34   MONTH / DAY / YEAR

S
M
T
W
T
F
S

Week 35   MONTH / DAY / YEAR

S
M
T
W
T
F
S

Week 36   MONTH / DAY / YEAR

S
M
T
W
T
F
S

HOW YOUR BABY IS GROWING

BY 36 WEEKS the baby is almost ready for birth, but still has to put on some fat to ensure that there is an efficient system for regulating heat and cold once she is outside the controlled environment of the uterus.

The baby is moving, blinking, passing urine, swallowing the amniotic fluid and hiccuping. Her muscles are strong, as you can feel from the vigorous kicking and thrusting of her arms and legs. If born at this time, the baby has an excellent chance of survival.

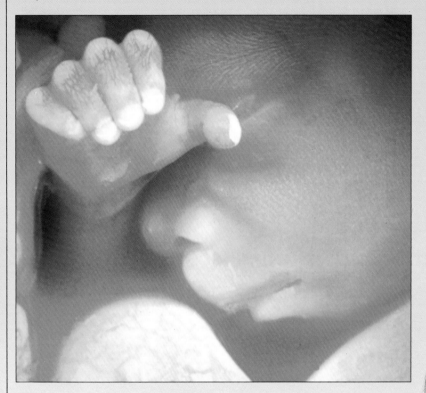

DOWNY HAIR *The baby's body may be covered with lanugo – fine, soft hair. This usually falls away before birth.*

The body is now plump, and approximately ¹/₂ oz (14 g) of fat is deposited under the skin every day.

Hair on the head can be up to 2 in (5 cm) long.

Did You Know

• The baby is nearly 18 in (45 cm) long from head to toe and weighs close on 6½ lb (3 kg). Boys may be a little heavier. From now, the rate of growth is much slower, but this is just as well: if the newborn baby continued to grow at the same rate as the fetus, she would weigh around 200 lb (90 kg) by her first birthday.

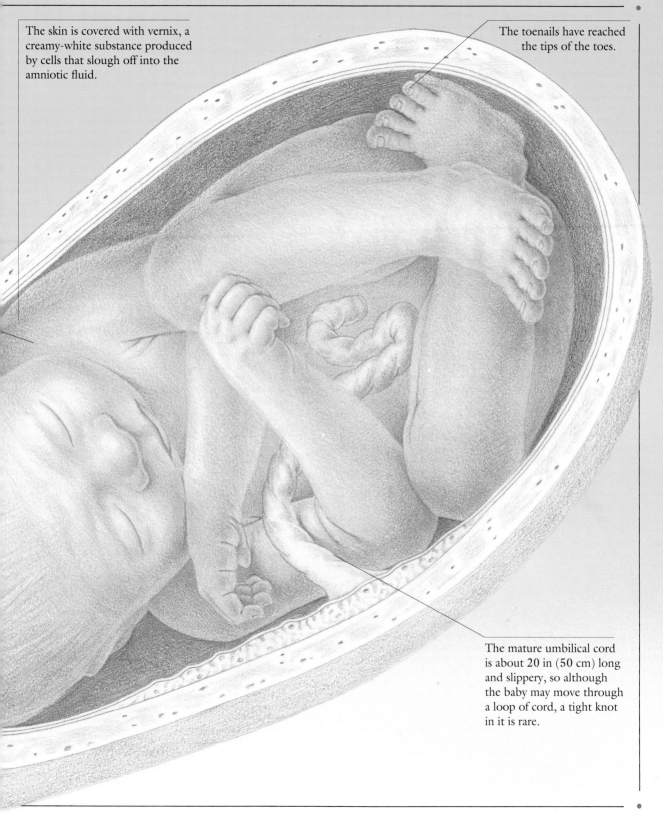

The skin is covered with vernix, a creamy-white substance produced by cells that slough off into the amniotic fluid.

The toenails have reached the tips of the toes.

The mature umbilical cord is about 20 in (50 cm) long and slippery, so although the baby may move through a loop of cord, a tight knot in it is rare.

HOW YOUR BABY IS LYING

A HEAD-DOWN POSITION is best for birth. A baby probably tips head-down in the last weeks of pregnancy because the head is its heaviest part. By this time most babies are lying on your left or right side with an ear towards your front. You can feel kicking on the side opposite to the baby's back. The feet and knees feel like knobs on an old-fashioned brass bed, and will move when you press them if the baby is awake. The buttocks feel pointed, like your bent elbow. You may be able to trace the firm curve of the baby's back.

~ CHANGES TO YOUR NAVEL ~

As the baby moves around, the shape of your abdomen and of your navel changes, too. When your baby is lying in a lateral or an anterior position (*see* right and below), you may find that your baby's back or shoulder makes your navel protrude. Some women find this area quite sensitive to touch. When your baby is in a posterior position (*see* page 99), your navel may lie in a saucer-like dip, which is the space between the baby's arms and legs.

~ LATERAL AND ANTERIOR POSITIONS ~

Before labor starts, the baby is often lying with an ear at the front – lateral – or the back of its head at the front – anterior. When it is lateral, Braxton-Hicks contractions (*see* page 70) nudge the baby around, so that by the time labor gets going the baby's back and the back of its head are usually towards your front. The exact position of the head is described in terms of the angle at which the crown, or occiput, is lying. This may be towards your front – anterior – or back – posterior. So, left occipito anterior is the crown of the head on the left at your front, and right occipito anterior is the crown of the head on the right at your front. These are the easiest positions for birth. The crown of the head fits snugly against your cervix, the spine is at the front, the arms and legs are bent, and everything is tucked in. The head is like a large ball, the body a smaller one. The neck allows these balls to turn in relation to each other, so as to take the curve of the birth canal.

Left occipito lateral (LOL)

Right occipito lateral (ROL)

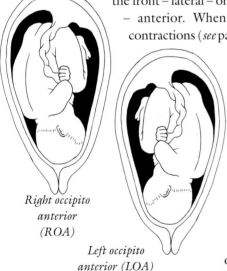

Right occipito anterior (ROA)

Left occipito anterior (LOA)

Back Labor

A backache is common in labor, especially if your baby is posterior. You can:

• Avoid lying on your back. Find positions in which you tilt the baby's weight off your spine: on all fours, kneeling, or leaning forward. Some big cushions will help you do this.
• Have firm hand pressure, a hot washcloth, hot water bottle, or heated picnic thermal pad on the place where your pelvis joins your spine.
• Have deep, firm, slow massage on the same spot.
• Rock your pelvis in a kneeling position, standing against a wall or in your partner's arms. If you are very tired, lie on your side.

~ OTHER POSITIONS ~

When a baby is posterior the spine lies against your back, so it is not as flexible to take the curve of the birth canal. The head may not be tucked into the chest. In labor you will feel the hard back of the baby's head pressing against your spine and get a backache. Most posterior babies turn to anterior before they are born, but it takes time, hours of back massage, patience – and a great deal of emotional support. Some babies get stuck in these positions and have to be helped out by forceps or vacuum extraction (*see* page 110).

The baby who is still bottom-down will probably be born as a breech. Occasionally a baby is transverse – lying horizontally across the uterus. Unless it is small and can be turned, it will not be able to get out like this, and will be born by Cesarean section (*see* page 111).

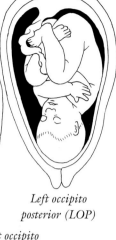

Left occipito posterior (LOP)

Right occipito posterior (ROP)

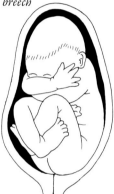

Flexed breech

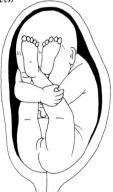

Frank breech

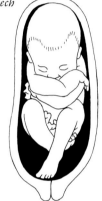

Footling breech

> *I didn't get the epidural we had planned because it was too fast. The second stage was two minutes. I felt something funny. I put down my hands and felt a foot sticking out. Then his body was born and I sat up to see his head delivered. I had no episiotomy and no stitches.*

FLEXED BREECH *The baby sits with its bottom over the cervix, its knees up to its abdomen, and sometimes with its legs crossed.*

FRANK BREECH *This is the commonest type of breech. The legs are straight, and the feet sometimes touch the ears. For a few days after birth, the legs will bounce back into this position.*

FOOTLING BREECH *This is rare but can happen especially with smaller babies. Either one or both feet are just above the cervix.*

TRACING YOUR BABY

Q In what different positions does your baby lie at this stage of pregnancy?

_____

_____

Q Can you feel your baby's feet, knees, buttocks, or spine?

_____

_____

TODAY'S DATE _____

FEEDING YOUR BABY

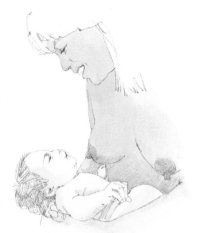

BREAST MILK is the best and natural food for babies. In its earliest form, colostrum, it is a concentrated food, particularly rich in protein, that provides protection for the baby against infections, too. So whether you decide that you want to feed the baby yourself or to use artificial milk, you will probably want to start by breastfeeding.

TUNING IN *Breastfeeding can help you get to know each other.*

~ GETTING STARTED ~

Some babies go straight to the breast like ducks to water. Others need to be encouraged and shown how to get a good latch. This happens with other animal babies, too. A mother cat nudges a kitten who is slow to catch on, and guides it to the source of food. So there is nothing wrong with you as a mother if learning about breastfeeding takes time.

LATCHING ON

The sucking reflex is very strong soon after birth, so the ideal time to put your baby to the breast first is within an hour and a half afterwards. Following that time, a baby may be sleepy and not at all interested. Start by getting yourself into a position that is comfortable for you and cuddling your baby close, so that she can smell, snuffle, and lick your bare skin.

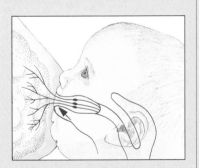

The baby presses the breast with a strong jaw . . .

Then "tease" her a little by touching her cheeks with your nipple.

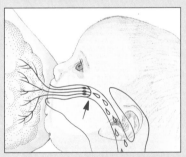

Her tongue presses the nipple against the roof of her mouth . . .

She gets excited, turns from side to side, opens her mouth wide, and latches on. Your baby needs to take in part or all of the dark circle around your nipple and to have a mouth full of breast. She can only pump the milk out when she can press on milk glands deep inside your breast. Then you can

see the jaw muscles above the ears working hard. If your nipples don't stand out, you can still get a good latch. As long as you give a generous mouthful of breast, your baby will mold the nipple to the right shape. If a breast is uncomfortably full and hard, express a little milk before feeding to soften it. Your midwife or a breastfeeding counselor will show you how to do this.

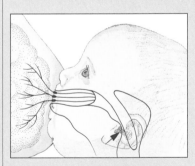

Milk spurts to the front of her mouth, and she swallows.

~ ROOMING-IN ~

Having your baby with you all the time, day and night, helps you both adapt to each other as in the steps of a dance. Feed your baby whenever she wants and for as long as she wants. This doesn't cause sore nipples. Not having the baby thoroughly latched on causes soreness.

~ HOW LONG AT EACH SIDE? ~

Let your baby suck as long as she wants at one side, then put her over your shoulder or hold her upright, leaning forward slightly, in your lap, and pat her back gently in case she has any air bubbles to bring up. When she seems ready to suck again, put her to your other breast and she will probably suck until she falls asleep. Sometimes she will have had enough milk at your first breast and won't need the other side. For the baby to obtain the rich, creamy milk that comes as the breast empties, it is important to have a good feeding at one side.

EASY BREASTFEEDING
You will need nursing bras but no special clothes, just T-shirts and sweaters.

He was a miserable, hungry baby. My nipples became sore, and I had a red, tender patch on my right breast. I phoned my breastfeeding counselor, who came over and explained that I was producing milk but it couldn't get out of my breasts because the baby wasn't on correctly. I had him lying so that he had to thrust his neck and turn his head. We were having a cup of tea at the time and she asked me to try drinking it like that. I couldn't of course. She showed me how to hold him with his legs under my arm, cradling his head with my hand. He latched on immediately and had a long, satisfying feeding."

"We're together in a milky wonderland."

"I couldn't give birth naturally, and it was very important that I could breastfeed. It's going well and has made up for the disappointment I felt about the birth.

THINKING ABOUT FEEDING

Q How do you feel about breastfeeding?

_____

_____

_____

_____

_____

_____

Q Who can you contact for help with breastfeeding?

_____

_____

_____

_____

TODAY'S DATE _____

BIRTH PARTNERS

A BIRTH PARTNER'S TASK is to give you emotional support and to focus entirely on you and your needs. The person you have chosen to share this most important experience with you may be the father of your baby, or a close friend or relative – man or woman. Whoever it is, your birth partner will be able to help you much better if he or she understands what will happen during labor and has prepared for the birth with you.

~ HELP IN THE FIRST STAGE ~

In the first stage, when your cervix is opening, you may begin to feel very tired and find it difficult to relax. To help you, your partner can sponge your face, breathe with you during difficult contractions, offer you sips of ice water, and encourage you to tune in to the rhythms of your body with each contraction. You may enjoy music, having lights dimmed, or being in darkness. Massage, and being stroked and held, can feel wonderful. You can walk or rock together. If you have back pain, firm counter-pressure in the small of your back feels good.

~ HELP IN TRANSITION ~

At this time your partner needs to be your anchor in a stormy sea of contractions. There is no place for doubt or fear. Then you move on to the second stage – the birth of your baby – with renewed energy and excitement.

UNDERSTANDING *Your birth partner needs to be aware of your feelings and to know how to give you strength.*

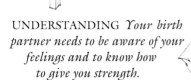

❝ *It was very important to me that Bill should be there all the time, and not leave me for anything. But we were told that fathers aren't allowed to be there for a forceps birth or a Cesarean and that they often get sent out during vaginal examinations. I felt my labor might just stop if that happened – so we changed hospitals.* ❞

EMPATHY *While rocking together, the same energy seems to flow through you both* (above).

FOCAL POINT *Ask your partner to concentrate entirely on you.*

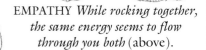

102

~ HELP IN THE SECOND STAGE ~

Now you get a passionate urge to push the baby out. Do this in any way that feels right for you. You may want your birth partner to hold you from behind in a semi-upright position, sitting or kneeling, for example, while your back is cradled against his or her body. If labor is progressing slowly, a supported squatting or standing position may help the baby down. As waves of power sweep through you, demanding all your energy to work with them, you may even forget that you are having a baby.

When the baby starts to move forward, your partner can suggest that you put your hands down and feel the top of the head. Then the head crowns, the forehead and face appear, and the head slips through. As the rest of the body slides out, you share the joy and wonder of the birth of your baby.

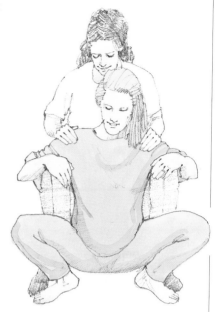

SUPPORT *Let your partner take your weight* (right).

TRUST *Relax and "ride" the pain together.*

> *The best thing of all was simply that he was there. Other people came and went, but he was always beside me."*

> "*My husband can't bear the sight of blood and he's nervous about anything to do with women's insides. I thought if he was there I'd be worrying all the time. Liz, my best friend, on the other hand, is stalwart, and she wanted to be there because she's training to be a birth educator and knows how to encourage you and support you physically. So she came — and we were a great team."*

REHEARSING FOR LABOR

Q What things are you and your birth partner practicing together in preparation for the birth?

_____

_____

_____

_____

Q What is the most important help your birth partner can give you during labor?

_____

_____

_____

_____

TODAY'S DATE _____

103

Weeks 37 *to* 40

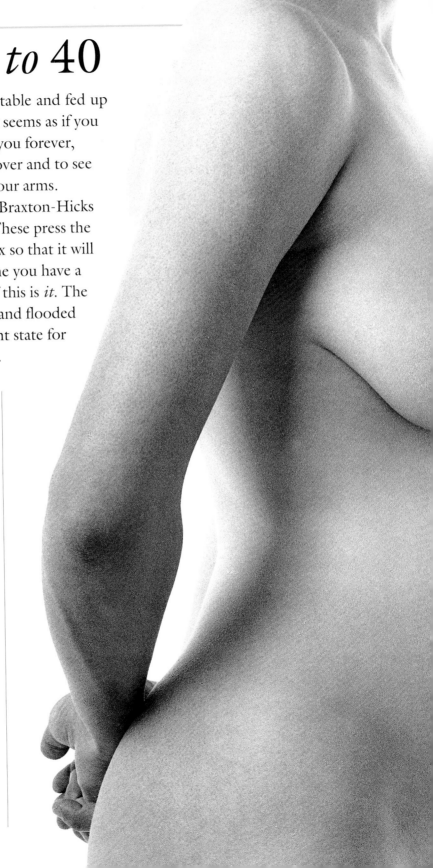

B Y NOW YOU MAY FEEL irritable and fed up with being pregnant. It seems as if you have had a baby inside you forever, and you long for it all to be over and to see and hold your baby in your arms.

You may be noticing more Braxton-Hicks contractions (*see* page 70). These press the baby's head against the cervix so that it will dilate more easily. Every time you have a cluster of them you wonder if this is *it*. The result is that you are excited and flooded with energy – in just the right state for the start of labor.

Body Facts

- You may have slight diarrhea.
- The baby's head feels like a coconut hanging between your legs and you have to remind yourself to tuck your bottom in and stand tall when you walk.
- You have a low backache.
- The top of the uterus may be lower now, because the baby has dipped into your pelvis, and you can breathe more easily.
- As your cervix starts to dilate a little, there is a blood-stained discharge from your vagina – the "show". It can occur a week or more before you actually go into labor.

I feel as if I have been pregnant for years. I'm tired, yet I can't sleep more than a couple of hours at a time. I can't wait to get this baby out!

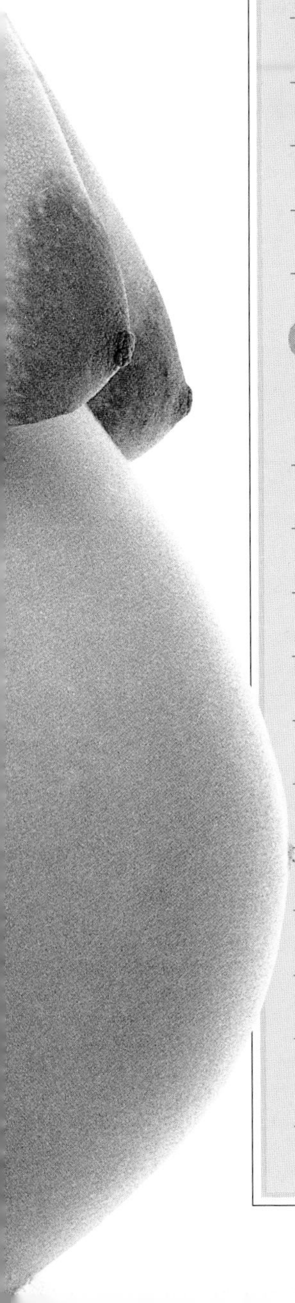

APPROACHING BIRTH

Q What are your feelings when you think about the birth?

_____

_____

_____

_____

_____

_____

Q Have you had any of the signs described in *Body Facts* that suggest that the birth is not far off?

_____

_____

_____

_____

_____

_____

_____

_____

_____

_____

_____

TODAY'S DATE _____

Week 37   MONTH / DAY / YEAR

S
M
T
W
T
F
S

Week 38   MONTH / DAY / YEAR

S
M
T
W
T
F
S

Week 39   MONTH / DAY / YEAR

S
M
T
W
T
F
S

Week 40   MONTH / DAY / YEAR

S
M
T
W
T
F
S

HOW YOUR BABY IS NOW

BY 37 WEEKS the baby's nervous system is maturing ready for birth. The layer of fat that has been building up under the skin is plump enough now for the baby to be able to regulate his body temperature when he is born.

It may be a tight fit in the uterus, so the baby is tucked up into a ball and can't make the big movements that you felt earlier. Instead of whole body rolls, you feel sharp kicks under your ribs at one side or the other.

The baby's lungs are lined with surfactant, which resembles bubbles of foam. When the baby is born, these bubbles keep the lungs partially inflated after each breath out. Without them, the lungs would collapse, the walls sticking together like plastic bags.

At birth it will be all systems go! So now the baby practices breathing movements, sucks and swallows, secretes enzymes and hormones ready for life outside, and has a whole range of co-ordinated reflexes that enable him to grasp tightly, lift and turn his head, find milk, make stepping movements, blink and close his eyes, and respond to sounds, smells, light, and touch.

When the baby's chin is well tucked in, the head will take the curve of the birth canal easily.

The head is not hard bone all over. There are soft gaps – the fontanelles – between the bones of the skull. As the baby slides down the birth canal, these can close up, molding the head for the journey.

A baby ready for birth weighs anything between 6 and 11 lb (2.9–5 kg). Its average length from crown to rump is approximately 14 in (35 cm).

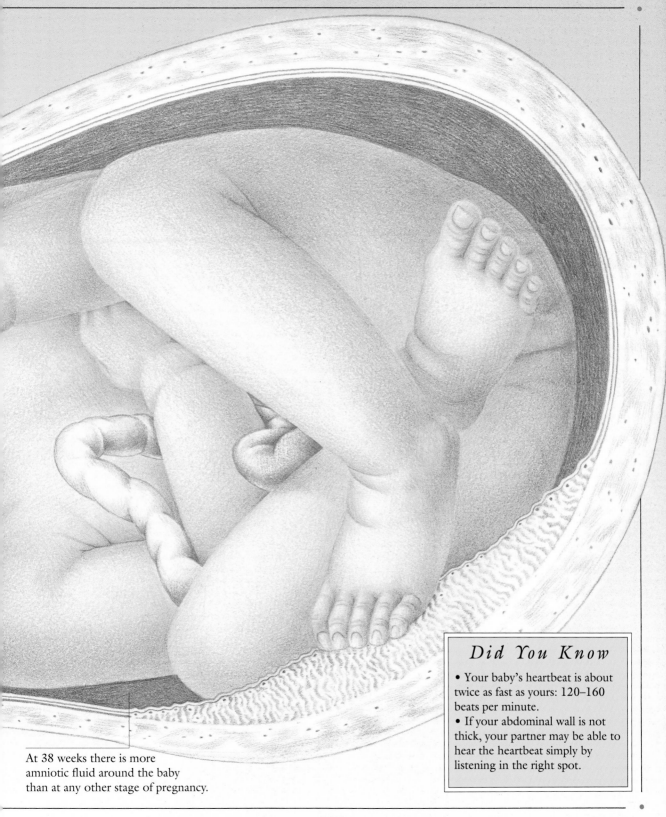

At 38 weeks there is more
amniotic fluid around the baby
than at any other stage of pregnancy.

Did You Know

• Your baby's heartbeat is about
twice as fast as yours: 120–160
beats per minute.
• If your abdominal wall is not
thick, your partner may be able to
hear the heartbeat simply by
listening in the right spot.

THE BIRTH

LABOR CAN START in three different ways. It may be with contractions like strong period pains. Or it may be a "show" – a blood-stained mucus discharge. Or your waters may break. But you can have a "show" as long as a week before labor begins, and waters may break hours before labor really gets going. When the contractions are more regular, contact your birth partner if he or she is not with you, and let friends who will be looking after your other children know. Now is a good time to check that you have everything you need: oil for massage, ice to suck, and anything that is comforting to have around you.

It was the most incredible experience. She was so beautiful as she gazed into my eyes. Tim couldn't stop crying. I felt so close to him."

"He slithered up on to my tummy. His eyes were incredibly bright, wide and open. I felt I'd known him for a long time.

AWAKE AND AWARE *A midwife supports the baby as the mother's hands reach down to lift the child from her body.*

~ EARLY FIRST STAGE ~

In the first stage your cervix opens. Do whatever feels intuitively right. You may find that you start to rock or sway during contractions, which gradually become more frequent, and stronger and longer. Take a bath or shower and let the sensation of water soothe you. Move around so that you can get into positions that are most comfortable for you.

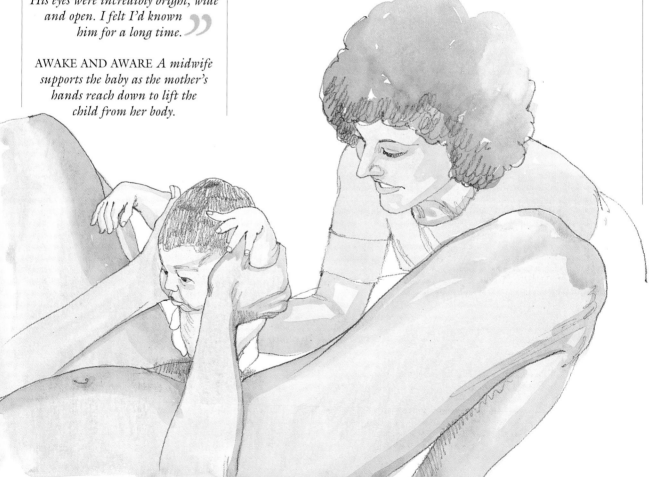

~ LATE FIRST STAGE ~

Contractions are now more intense, and flow through you like ocean waves. You will be using a great deal of energy. You may find that you relax more fully if you have an inner focus and vivid pictures in your mind of what is happening inside you. There will be pain-relieving drugs if you need them. Explore different positions that feel comfortable, and ask your partner to rub your back. Take one contraction at a time, breathing your way carefully through each.

Nausea and sickness may be a problem now, and you can suck ice cubes to keep your mouth fresh. Your body produces endorphins – nature's own painkillers – which help you relax and make you more focused. It may seem as if the encouraging words of your midwife and other helpers are coming from far away.

~ TRANSITION ~

This is a short but intense time. Contractions become more painful, you may get an urge to push, and think that you cannot cope much longer. You may get irritable with your partner, want labor to stop, and feel very emotional. Just before the onset of the second stage, many women have a peaceful and refreshing lull.

I was as interested in her as I might be in a puppy or kitten, but I didn't feel she belonged to me. They took her off so that the pediatrician could have a look at her. Six hours later they brought her to me all wrapped up and told me I should feed her. I needed help, but the nurses were too busy. Neither of us knew what to do.

~ SECOND STAGE ~

After the cervix has opened completely, you begin to have an involuntary urge to push at the height of contractions. You may feel that you want to open your bowels, as the baby presses on to the nerves that give you this sensation. The feeling of wanting to push deep into your bottom gradually becomes overwhelming, and heralds the second stage.

An upright, kneeling, or squatting position is best for the second stage, as your pushing efforts are helped by gravity. You and your uterus work together to move your baby further down into your vagina. You let yourself open wider and wider, and at last . . . your baby!

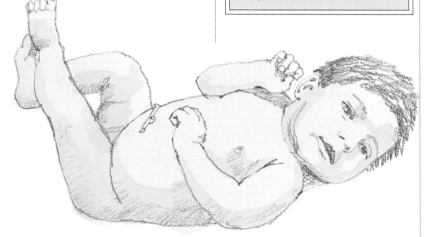

What is the Third Stage?

• The third stage of labor is the separation and delivery of the placenta and membranes.

• When the baby is born, the uterus continues to contract, and the placenta separates from the uterine wall.

• You can push the placenta out yourself. Squatting is best for doing this.

• Putting your baby to the breast helps the uterus contract.

• In most hospitals this process is speeded up by an injection of the hormone oxytocin, which makes the uterus contract more quickly. The midwife or doctor then pulls on the cord to deliver the placenta and membranes.

ALERT AND WIDE-EYED
A baby starts to discover his new world from the moment of birth.

She was covered in vernix which was sticking all over her like a facepack. But she was beautiful. It took her about eight seconds to breathe and then she took a big gasp and turned pink. She was wide awake.

HELPING THE BABY OUT

I F IT TAKES A LONG TIME to push the baby out, if changes in the heart-rate indicate that the baby is over-stressed, if your blood pressure rises or if you get exhausted, the simplest way of speeding the birth may be an episiotomy – cut – to enlarge the birth opening. But many episiotomies are done unnecessarily. If the baby is not very near birth, you may be moved to a delivery room, so that an obstetrician can help the baby out with a forceps delivery or vacuum extraction. You have the right to be fully informed of this and to be involved in all the discussion and any decisions being made.

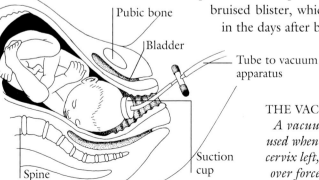

Pubic bone

Bladder

Forceps

Spine

A STRONG PULL *Forceps clasp the baby's head and draw it down and forward. The strength of pull in a forceps delivery is like that needed to get a very tight cork out of a wine bottle.*

“ *We'd talked about forceps births at our classes, and like everyone else I didn't think it would happen to me. Despite all my pushing she wouldn't budge, so I had forceps. The doctor did a small episiotomy, as she knew I hadn't really wanted one.* ”

~ EPISIOTOMY ~

A local anesthetic is given in the perineum – the tissues around your vagina – and a cut made with scissors through skin and muscle at the lower end of the vagina. It is stitched up again after the birth. Ask for more local anesthetic if you need it. In **20 percent** of women, an episiotomy extends into a severe tear, so it is worth avoiding.

~ FORCEPS ~

Forceps are like metal salad tongs with a hinge in the handle. Your legs are raised in stirrups. Ask to have two or three pillows under your head and shoulders so that you can catch the first glimpse of your baby. If the area is not already anesthetized, you are given a local anesthetic so that you are ready for an episiotomy if you need one. Then the blades of the forceps are inserted and cupped around the sides of the baby's head. The doctor pulls and you push together. You can ask to have the forceps taken off once the head is born, so that you can push the rest of the baby out yourself.

~ VACUUM EXTRACTION ~

A vacuum extractor works like a miniature vacuum cleaner, and can be used without an episiotomy. A suction cup is placed on the baby's head and the baby is sucked out with each contraction as you push. This produces a bump on the head like a large, bruised blister, which gradually subsides in the days after birth.

Pubic bone

Bladder

Tube to vacuum apparatus

Suction cup

Spine

THE VACUUM EXTRACTOR
A vacuum extractor can be used when there is still a rim of cervix left, so has an advantage over forceps, which cannot be used in this way.

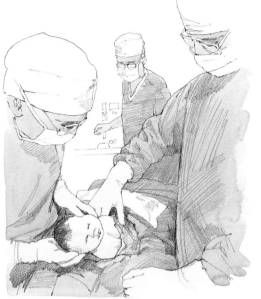

TIME TO RECOVER

A Cesarean section is a major operation from which you will need time to recuperate.

> *I had an emergency Cesarean last time after many hours of labor. This time I decided to have an epidural Cesarean. I didn't feel a thing. Robert was able to hold him right away.*

~ CESAREAN SECTION ~

A Cesarean is a planned (elective), or an emergency procedure that is done because there is risk to the baby, or sometimes to you. It may be the only way to have a safe birth if the placenta is lying in front of the head, or if the mother has severe pre-eclampsia (*see* page 92). Although some doctors perform one whenever a cervix is slow to dilate, and for all breech babies, this is not essential, and means that many unnecessary Cesareans are done.

If you have had a Cesarean before, this does not mean that you need have one next time. Each labor is different. Many women who have had a Cesarean go on to have vaginal births if they are free to move around, take their own time, and have strong emotional support.

~ EPIDURAL OR GENERAL ANESTHESIA? ~

If you have a Cesarean birth, you may have the choice between an epidural or general anesthesia. If you would like your partner to stay with you, make this clear, although it may not be allowed if you have general anesthesia. With an epidural you can ask to take a tape recorder into the delivery room and for ceiling lights to be dimmed. You can see and even hold your baby immediately. After general anesthesia, most women feel groggy. But when a decision is made during labor to do a Cesarean section, there may be no time for an epidural. If you have general anesthesia, you can ask if your partner can cuddle the baby before you wake up. The baby may have been taken to the nursery by the time you are awake. Your partner can go there to be with her and, as soon as you feel able, you can ask to be wheeled to meet your baby.

YOUR SPECIAL WISHES

Q What are your special wishes if you have a forceps delivery or vacuum extraction?

_____

_____

_____

_____

TODAY'S DATE _____

Q What are your special wishes if you have a Cesarean section?

_____

_____

_____

_____

BEING OVERDUE

ONCE PAST YOUR DUE DATE, every day seems like a week, every week like a month. Each twinge alerts you to the possible start of labor, and you become hypersensitive to Braxton-Hicks contractions – the "rehearsal" contractions of the uterus that you may feel like firm squeezes of your whole abdomen. Many women have "false labor" because they so much want to start. Some women feel under threat of induction, too. Suddenly everything seems to become abnormal, and you are supposed to let doctors take over.

GETTING READY
An intravenous drip of Pitocin means that you can't move about freely, so get really comfortable before it is set up.

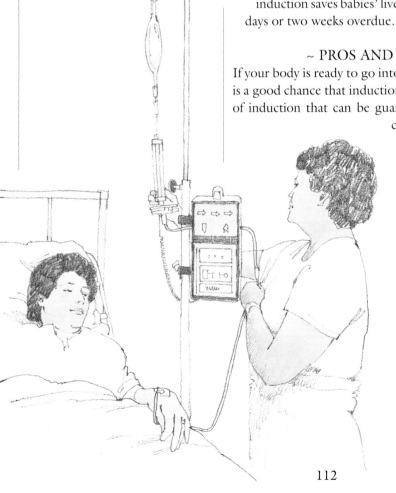

~ WHAT IS INDUCTION? ~

Induction means starting labor artificially. It is not always successful. The most common reason for induction of labor is that a woman is overdue. It may entail stripping the membranes and puncturing the bag of waters with an instrument that looks like a crochet hook. Or an intravenous drip of Pitocin, a synthetic form of the hormone oxytocin, may be set up. Sometimes both approaches are used. There is no evidence that induction saves babies' lives when it is done simply because labor is ten days or two weeks overdue.

~ PROS AND CONS OF INDUCTION ~

If your body is ready to go into labor and your cervix is already ripe, there is a good chance that induction will be successful. But there is no method of induction that can be guaranteed to be both absolutely certain and completely safe.

Artificial rupture of the membranes has disadvantages because it means that the protective bubble in which the baby lies is gone. The release of Pitocin in an I.V. must be carefully controlled, or you may have a labor that is fast, furious, and painful. Both of these methods may increase the need for an assisted delivery, too, with forceps or vacuum extraction, or for a Cesarean section.

If induction is proposed, you can say you want to discuss it fully beforehand, ask exactly why it is recommended for you, and find out what form it will take. You do not have to agree to induction if you find the reasons unconvincing. If you do go ahead and have labor induced, you will need very good emotional support from a confident birth companion.

STIMULATING LABOR YOURSELF

If you feel that you are under pressure to accept induction, and want to keep control of your body, there are some things you can try for yourself to help start labor.

~ BREAST MASSAGE ~
Stroking your breasts gently and stimulating your nipples releases natural oxytocin into your bloodstream. This helps your cervix ripen and may even start labor. If your breasts are very full and tender, you may want to massage them yourself. Or your partner may like to do this for you. You may need to massage your breasts for up to an hour three times in each 24 hours.

~ MAKING LOVE ~
Any kind of love-making, provided that you enjoy it, stimulates oxytocin release, too. It should be slow and sensuous. Have the room warm, and see that you will be undisturbed. The "spoons" position – where

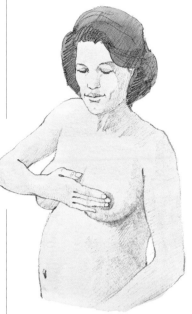

STROKING YOUR NIPPLES
You can stimulate the release of oxytocin by doing this.

at the same time, too. But lying on your back with your partner above you enables semen, which is rich in natural prostaglandins that cause the uterus to contract, to soak into your cervix.

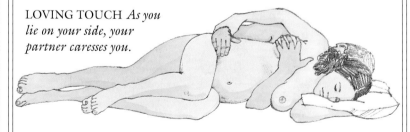

LOVING TOUCH *As you lie on your side, your partner caresses you.*

you nestle with your back against the front of your partner's body – will probably be the most comfortable, and your partner will be able to stimulate your breasts

If you begin to have contractions every two minutes or less, reduce or stop the stimulation, as things may be moving too fast for you, or for the baby's comfort.

"I was three days past my expected date and went to the receptionist's desk to arrange admission for induction at the end of the week – since the consultant told me that I must as it was hospital policy – and she said, 'We are very busy then, come in now.' I was very shaken."

"I was 39 weeks and the doctor said, 'I guarantee no more than a ten-hour labor. When do you want to have your baby?'"

"When I was 36 weeks he told me that labor would be induced. I said that the baby wasn't due, so why, and he said there was uncertainty about the date of my last period. I was very upset and asked more questions. He agreed I was very fit, and said it was because the placenta gets old if the baby is overdue, and that if I wanted to go full term it was at my own risk. I said I was prepared to accept that risk. Labor started naturally at 40 weeks, there were no problems, and the baby is fine."

"The doctor said that induction was very likely to be successful because my cervix was ripe already and the baby was deeply engaged. In fact, I was two centimeters dilated without knowing it. Contractions started coming at five-minute intervals. I phoned Jim to tell him to come in, and, soon after he arrived, I went straight into contractions at two-minute intervals. They were tough to handle, but Jim breathed with me through each one, just like we had practiced together. She was born as the sun rose on a lovely summer's day."

ACTIVE BIRTH

IT USED TO BE THOUGHT that the proper place for a woman to have a baby was in bed where she was treated as if she were ill. Even today many people assume that this is natural. It isn't, of course. In many traditional cultures women keep moving during childbirth. The advantages of being upright and mobile – and having an active birth – are being rediscovered now: the woman feels more in control, contractions are more efficient, pain is reduced, labor is shorter, and the baby is in better condition than when the mother is flat on her back. If you want an active birth, it helps to learn stretching and opening movements, many of which are derived from yoga, and to move rhythmically, rock your pelvis, and make any noises you want. You don't have to put on an exhibition – just be free to do whatever you feel like doing. You will then be able to work *with* your body instead of fighting it. You will know exactly what movements and positions can relieve pain, and how to make your pelvis wide to let the baby through.

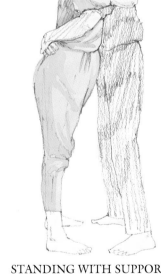

STANDING WITH SUPPORT
Like this you can do a slow, rolling belly-dance together.

❝ *Standing was best, and I lunged forward with my hands on the wall when the contractions came.* ❞

~ MOVING IN THE FIRST STAGE ~

Through the long hours of the first stage, it helps to avoid getting stuck in one position, and to keep moving. You greet each contraction with slow, full breathing, using your helpers and furniture in the room for physical support. Your birth attendants rock and move gently with you, subtly adapting to the rhythm of your contractions. This enables you to breathe without strain, and allows your cervix to open.

Standing positions with feet wide apart, and knees unlocked and slightly bent, feel good. You may want to walk around, leaning against a wall or your partner when a contraction comes. Some women like something to hold on to, from which they can hang – such as a towel draped over a hook that is attached firmly to the ceiling or a wall, or a helper's neck.

If you have a backache, you will want to find positions in which you tip the baby on to your abdominal wall, and where your partner can offer strong counter-pressure or massage on each side of your lower spine. Forward-leaning, kneeling, or all-fours positions are best for this.

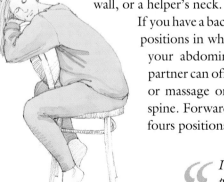

SITTING *Leaning over the back of a chair is often comfortable.*

❝ *I liked leaning over a pillow on a birth stool, with my belly over the curve of the stool, and I rocked and circled my pelvis.* ❞

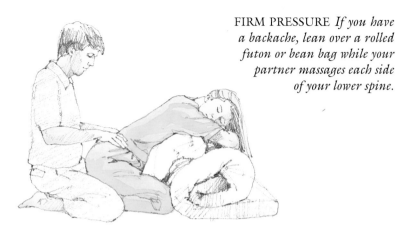

FIRM PRESSURE *If you have a backache, lean over a rolled futon or bean bag while your partner massages each side of your lower spine.*

~ MOVING IN THE SECOND STAGE ~

In a squatting, kneeling, or half-kneeling/half-squatting position your pelvic floor muscles are released and stretched, and open more easily. Make sure that your inner thigh muscles are relaxed, and that when you push you can move the small of your back, round your shoulders, and let your head drop forward. Having help from someone who adapts their posture and movement to your spontaneous pushing, while providing solid support, may be better than using special equipment.

Many women like to be able to get their feet flat on the ground, and push most effectively, and relax the perineum best in one of these positions. If you choose to give birth in a standing squat with your helper behind you, it is better for him or her to grasp your wrists or forearms than to grip under your arms, since that can cause temporary nerve damage in your arms if done for a long time.

SQUATTING *Your pelvis is at its widest in this position.*

" I did pelvic tilting and rocking, and it was much better than last time when I got stuck in one position with a terrible backache. I pushed on my knees, leaning over the headboard of the bed. Having my hips free really helped. Our 11-pound son was born after just over an hour in the second stage, sliding out easily into the midwife's hands – and I didn't even tear."

"It wasn't an easy or pain-free birth, but I can honestly say I enjoyed it. Being able to move was very important to me. In classes I practiced unlocking my knees and pelvic joints, and when it came to it I could go along with the contractions, like getting into the beat of music. "

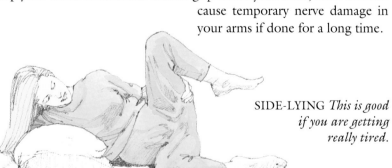

SIDE-LYING *This is good if you are getting really tired.*

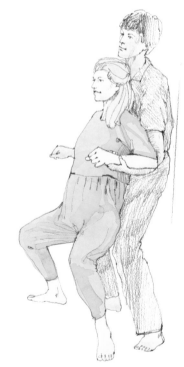

STANDING SQUAT *In this position gravity helps as you push, and your helper takes your weight.*

WATER IN CHILDBIRTH

WATER IS SOOTHING and helps you to relax. It is easy to move freely in water, and the very idea of water – comforting, flowing, streaming onwards – encourages you to think of your body opening. This may have a powerful physiological effect, enable your cervix to open, and help you to accept the power welling up in your body.

TAKING A SHOWER
Water streaming over your body can feel wonderful.

❝ The midwife and I walked around the garden in the first stage. I squatted down holding on to a tree when contractions came. By the time I was seven centimeters dilated it seemed a long way between trees! I longed to be in the water, so I jumped in, and it was wonderful! I refused to get out after that, and the baby was born very slowly and gently under the water and came up into my arms.❞

"My obstetrician put a step stool in the pool for the delivery of my breech baby. He had forceps but didn't need to use them. ❞

~ BATH OR SHOWER ~

The simplest way of using water during labor is to lie and soak in a warm bath. Have the water as deep as possible. The buoyancy of water counteracts the effects of gravity, and helps you to relax, let go of your inhibitions, and surrender to the natural rhythms of your body.

While you are lying in the bath you can pour or trickle water from a jug over your abdomen as each contraction builds to a peak, or ask your partner to do this for you. Bathroom lighting is usually bright, so you may prefer candlelight. In hospital, where a bath may not be available, you may like to stand – or squat on a stool – under a shower and let warm water pour over you. If a helper is going to get into a shower or birth pool with you, it is a good idea to pack his swimming trunks or her swimsuit in your suitcase.

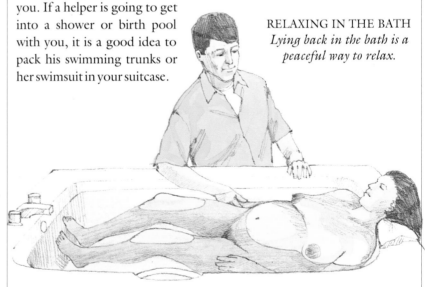

RELAXING IN THE BATH
Lying back in the bath is a peaceful way to relax.

~ HELPING A BACK LABOR ~

If the baby is lying in a posterior position, you may have back labor. Sitting under a shower, or having a helper sponge warm water gently over your back as each contraction increases in intensity can help reduce pain. In a deep bath or pool you can kneel or be on all fours, so that the hard back of the baby's head is tilted slightly away from your lower spine. Because it provides a counter-stimulus to pain, a strong jet of water from a hand-held shower directed on to the area of greatest discomfort gives amazing relief.

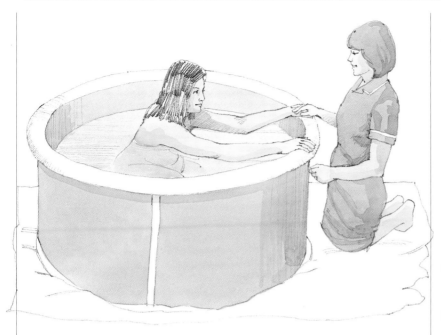

~ WATERBIRTH IN A POOL ~

A birth pool is a deep, round tank lined with plastic and filled with warm water, where you can float during labor. The top edge is usually padded, so that it is soft for you to lean against, and the water temperature may be thermostatically controlled. Some birth centers and a few hospitals have pools, and you can also rent – or even buy – one for use at home.

Women who use birth pools often like to labor in warm water, but want to have their feet on solid ground to push the baby out. Others like to stay in the water and give birth there. Whatever feels right for you at the time is the best thing to do.

Other Ways of Using Water

• A soft washcloth or a natural sponge soaked in warm or cool water (whichever feels better) can be squeezed out and used as a compress on your back, abdomen, face, or neck.
• An ice pack cools your face and neck if you're feeling hot and irritable.
• Suck ice cubes if you don't feel like drinking.
• A non-aerosol spray of water or plant spray refreshes you.

• A baby's hot-water bottle, or a picnic thermal pack heated up in warm water and wrapped in a small, soft towel is soothing if you need continuous warmth, or to rest against your lower abdomen or between your legs.
• A miniature natural sponge dipped in ice water is ideal for moistening your lips.
• Ice water in a vacuum flask, if a supply is not available, can be used with a sponge or washcloth.

MAKING YOUR OWN SPACE
If you are in a birth pool, it may be best not to have your helpers in the water with you, so that you have your own private space and can move freely. The midwife may appreciate a bean bag, big floor cushion, or padded stool on which to kneel to prevent her from straining her back.

I didn't sink down in the water. I enjoyed moving. I felt my body tell me what to do – what I needed to do for me and the baby. So I crouched and turned and plunged and kicked. It felt just right!

"I really wanted a bath in the delivery suite since I'd found them so comforting at home. Once I was in the bath my contractions became much more intense and I just couldn't move. So I gave birth to her there. The midwife and I laughed afterwards because one side of her hair was wet where she'd been listening with the fetoscope."

"In transition it got very tough and the pain was continuous. I wanted to give up, and Stewart was obviously tired. I had a woman friend with me too. She came in under the shower and we danced and sang and moaned together, while Stewart lay on the bed and talked to the midwife! When I came out of the shower I was fully dilated.

GENTLE BIRTH

HAVE YOU THOUGHT what it may feel like to be born? Some births are violent for both mother and baby. Yet even a birth that is a happy experience for the parents may entail violence to a baby. The newborn may be handled and examined without sensitivity and with quick, rough movements, exposed to bright lights, startled by loud voices, then be more or less isolated from human contact in a plastic box and put in a nursery with other crying babies.

~ MOMENTS BEFORE BIRTH ~

You can choose to give birth in an upright or semi-upright position, so that you can see from the first moments when only the top of the baby's head is visible. Having a mirror helps, and if you ask someone to hold it at a slant over your lower abdomen, you can watch the head moving forward.

If you put your hand down, you can stroke the warm, firm bulge of your baby's head even before it is born. Then the head slides out and turns so that you can see the face, and the shoulders and whole body are born.

Before the baby slips out, lights can be turned down. In dim light or in darkness she is more likely to open her eyes and look at you.

What the Baby Feels

- The baby probably feels even strong contractions as hugs.
- The opening cervix is usually firmly cupped against the back of the baby's head.
- As the baby is pressed down, the head and body are squeezed into a tighter ball. If this squeezing is very marked, blood-flow to the brain is reduced at the height of contractions, and the baby feels nothing for a few moments.

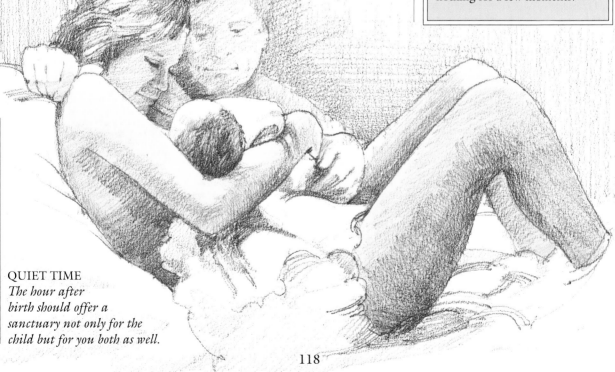

QUIET TIME
The hour after birth should offer a sanctuary not only for the child but for you both as well.

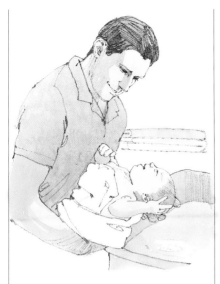

LEBOYER BATH *Some parents like to bathe their baby soon after birth, so that the newborn can discover her limbs in the familiar environment of water.*

"*We considered the Leboyer bath. I think it's a lovely idea for the father to bathe his baby. But when it came to it, our little boy was so contented at the breast that we decided to put off the bath until the next day. We both enjoyed doing it then.*"

"*In my Birth Plan I asked for dim lights. In the end I had to have low forceps because she got stuck. Even so, the doctor respected my wishes, and the main room lights were switched off, with just a spotlight so that he could see what he was doing. He said, 'Good, there's the widest part of the head through. Why don't you push the rest of the baby out yourself?' So I did, and lifted her up, warm and slithery and wet, into my arms. It was an unforgettable moment!*"

~ ENTERING THE WORLD ~

Slowly, gently, the baby is drawn up on to your abdomen or over your thigh. You hold her right away, and, as she lies against your body, can feel the throbbing in the cord with your hand. Ask the doctor or midwife to wait for the cord to stop pulsating before clamping and cutting it, and to delay any injection of oxytocin that would force blood into the baby's circulation. Request that a catheter (a fine tube) be put in the baby's mouth and nose to suck out mucus only if she needs it.

In some hospitals there is a bustle of activity and a rush to deliver the placenta, clear things away, and clean up. A newborn baby is startled by loud voices and clattering equipment, so ask for a quiet, tranquil setting.

Rest the baby against your bare breast. After a while she will seek the nipple and may lick it first. When she is ready to suck she opens her mouth, and you put her to your breast for the first nursing.

A baby hears and responds to its mother's voice, so talk to her. Knowing what to say will come naturally. Ask to have extended time together in peace before being moved. Hold, cuddle, and caress your baby as much as you like, keeping her close beside you. It is a good start to life for the baby and a good beginning for all of you as a family.

WELCOMING YOUR BABY

Q What things would you like to do to welcome your baby into the world?

_____

_____

_____

_____

_____

_____

_____

_____

_____

_____

TODAY'S DATE _____

THE MOMENTS AFTER BIRTH

Y OU REACH OUT to take your baby in your arms, and at last gaze at each other face to face. Most babies explore their mother's face and make eye contact within a few minutes of birth. Welcome your baby with skin-to-skin touch. Let him know that your body is a safe haven. When he starts to root around, put him to the breast. However tiring labor has been, most women are on a high for the first hours after birth, if the baby is with them.

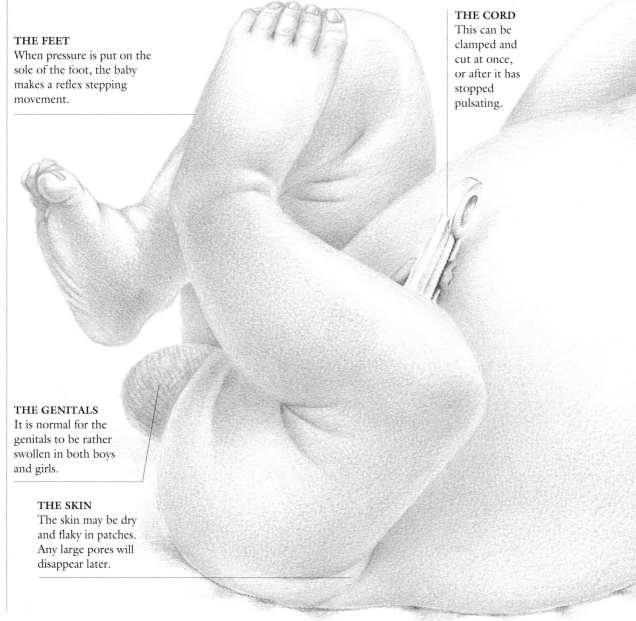

THE FEET
When pressure is put on the sole of the foot, the baby makes a reflex stepping movement.

THE CORD
This can be clamped and cut at once, or after it has stopped pulsating.

THE GENITALS
It is normal for the genitals to be rather swollen in both boys and girls.

THE SKIN
The skin may be dry and flaky in patches. Any large pores will disappear later.

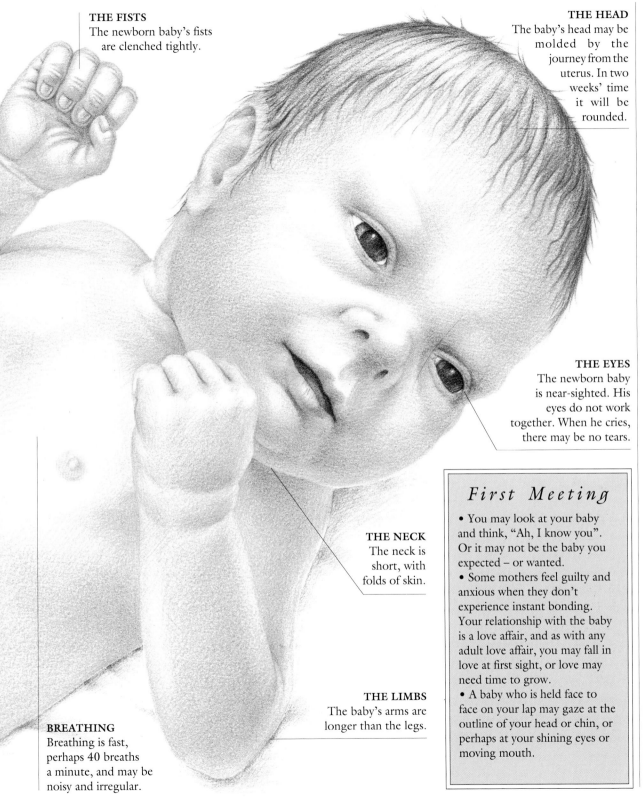

THE FISTS
The newborn baby's fists are clenched tightly.

THE HEAD
The baby's head may be molded by the journey from the uterus. In two weeks' time it will be rounded.

THE EYES
The newborn baby is near-sighted. His eyes do not work together. When he cries, there may be no tears.

THE NECK
The neck is short, with folds of skin.

THE LIMBS
The baby's arms are longer than the legs.

BREATHING
Breathing is fast, perhaps 40 breaths a minute, and may be noisy and irregular.

First Meeting

• You may look at your baby and think, "Ah, I know you". Or it may not be the baby you expected – or wanted.
• Some mothers feel guilty and anxious when they don't experience instant bonding. Your relationship with the baby is a love affair, and as with any adult love affair, you may fall in love at first sight, or love may need time to grow.
• A baby who is held face to face on your lap may gaze at the outline of your head or chin, or perhaps at your shining eyes or moving mouth.

YOUR BIRTH ACCOUNT

THESE PAGES ARE FOR YOU to tell the story of your baby's birth in your own words. Events that are vividly in your mind now can fade or change as time goes by. You may want to remember exactly what happened so that you can tell your child about how he or she came into the world. You can begin by telling how labor started, where you were and what you were doing. At the end, you can describe how you felt when you first held your baby in your arms.

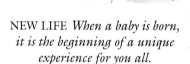

NEW LIFE *When a baby is born, it is the beginning of a unique experience for you all.*

Your Photographs

BOOKS AND RESOURCES

Heart & Hands: A Midwife's Guide to Pregnancy and Birth, 3rd ed.
Davis, Elizabeth
  Celestial Arts, 1997

Birthing from Within: An Extra-Ordinary Guide to Childbirth Preparation
England, Pam and Rob Horowitz
  Partera Press, 1998

Spiritual Midwifery, 3rd ed.
Gaskin, Ina May
  The Book Publishing Company, 1990

Gentle Birth Choices
Harper, Barbara
  Inner Traditions International, Ltd., 1994
Available with or without 47-minute video showing several different births.

Becoming a Grandmother
Kitzinger, Sheila
  Fireside, 1997

Breastfeeding Your Baby, rev. ed.
Kitzinger, Sheila
  Knopf, 1998

The Complete Book of Pregnancy and Childbirth, rev. ed.
Kitzinger, Sheila
  Knopf, 1996

Rediscovering Birth
Kitzinger, Sheila
  Pocket Books, 2000

The Year After Childbirth
Kitzinger, Sheila
  Fireside, 1996

Your Baby and Child, rev. ed.
Leach, Penelope
  Knopf, 1997

Easing Labor Pain
Lieberman, Adrienne
  Harvard Common Press, 1992

Nine Months and a Day
Lieberman, Adrienne
  Harvard Common Press, 2000

When a Baby Dies: A Handbook for Healing and Helping, rev. ed.
Limbo, Rana K. and Sara Rich Wheeler
  Lutheran Hospital/Lacrosse, 1998

Women Giving Birth
Limburg, Astrid and Beatrijs Smulders
  Celestial Arts, 1993

Essential Exercises for the Childbearing Year, 4th ed.
Noble, Elizabeth
  New Life Images, 1995

Birth Reborn
Odent, Michael
  Birth Works, 1994

The Tentative Pregnancy: How Amniocentesis Changes the Experience of Motherhood
Rothman, Barbara Katz
  Norton, 1993

After the Tears: Parents Talk about Raising a Child with a Disability
Simons, Robin
  Harcourt Brace Jovanovich, 1987

Special Delivery: Creating the Birth You Want for You and Your Baby
Baldwin, Rahima
  1988. VHS, 42 minutes, $44.95
Available from International Childbirth Education Association.
Emphasizes parents' responsibility for choosing the birth suited to them. Shows three births: in a hospital; a birth center; at home.

Midwifery Today
Magazine available in print or online:
  www.midwiferytoday.com

USEFUL ORGANIZATIONS

American Academy of Husband-Coached Childbirth (AAHCC)
(Bradley Method)
P.O. Box 5224
Sherman Oaks, CA 91413
(818) 788-6662 or (800) 4ABIRTH
www.bradleybirth.com

American College of Nurse-Midwives (ACNM)
818 Connecticut Ave., N.W.
Suite 900
Washington, D.C. 20006
(202)728-9860; fax (202)728-9897
www.midwife.com

Birth and Life Bookstore
Cascade Health Care Products
141 Commercial Street, N.E.
Salem, OR 97301
(503) 371-4445
www.1cascade.com

International Cesarean Awareness Network (ICAN)
1304 Kingsdale Avenue
Redondo Beach, CA 90278
(310)542-6400; fax (310)542-5368
www.childbirth.org/ICAN/

Cesareans/Support, Education and Concern (C/SEC)
22 Forest Road
Framingham, MA 01701
(508) 877-8266

The Compassionate Friends
P.O. Box 3696
Oak Brook, IL 60522-3696
(630)990-0010; fax (630)990-0246
www.compassionatefriends.org
Helps those who have suffered a perinatal bereavement.

Association of Labor Assistants and Childbirth Educators (ALACE)
(formerly Informed Home Birth)
P.O. Box 382724
Cambridge, MA 02238
(617) 441-2500
server4.hypermart.net/alacehq/

International Childbirth Education Association (ICEA)
P.O. Box 20048
Minneapolis, MN 55420-0048
(952)854-8660 or (800)624-4934
www.icea.org

La Leche League International (LLLI)
1400 N. Meacham
Schaumburg, IL 60173-4048
(847)519-7730 or (800)LALECHE
www.lalecheleague.org

Lamaze International
(ASPO/Lamaze)
2025 M Street, N.W.
Suite 800
Washington, D.C. 20036-3309
(800)368-4404 or (202)367-1128
www.lamaze-childbirth.com

Maternity Center Association
281 Park Ave South, 5th Floor,
New York, NY 10128
(212) 777-5000;
fax (212) 777-9320
www.maternity.org

National Association of Childbearing Centers (NACC)
3123 Gottschall Road
Perkiomenville, PA 18074
(215)234-8068; fax (215)234-8829
www.birthcenters.org
Maintains a list of birthing centers.

National Women's Health Network
514 10th Street, N.W.
Suite 400
Washington, D.C. 20004
(202)347-1140; fax (202)347-1168
www.womenshealthnetwork.org

Planned Parenthood Federation of America, Inc.
810 Seventh Avenue
New York, NY 10019
(212)541-7800 or (800)230-7526
www.plannedparenthood.org

Women, Infants & Children Supplementary Food Program (WIC)
Contact your State Department of Health for local office.

INDEX

~ ACKNOWLEDGMENTS ~

The authors would like to thank Uwe and David for their love and encouragement. Vital secretarial skills were provided by Judith Schroeder, Kim Hamilton, and David Bailey. Both of us want to thank the midwives with whom we work, and the mothers who have contributed so much to these pages. Claire and Richard Carlton became the proud parents of Jude while we were writing this book. Special thanks to Vic and Mary Hazel, Alison Hazel, Lorna Warren, Fran Dutton, Janice Williams, Jackie Couves, Naomi Morton, and Betty Angus. Daphne Maurer's and Charles Maurer's book *The World of the Newborn* (Viking 1988) provided us with a rich source of material on the behavior of the baby in the uterus, for which we are grateful. We would also like to thank the National Childbirth Trust for the quotations from mothers with disabilities on pages 50 and 51, selected (in abbreviated form) from "The Emotions and Experiences of Some Disabled Mothers" (National Childbirth Trust 1985).

Dorling Kindersley would like to thank the staff at Richmond for help with artwork references; Kate Grant for initial inputting of text; Rosalind Priestley and Maryann Rogers for help with production; and Janos Marffy for airbrushing. **Special photography** by Nancy Durrell McKenna on pages 26–27, 38–39, 52–53, 74–75, 84–85, 94–95, 104–105. **Photographs** by Nancy Durrell McKenna on page 8; by Lennart Nilsson on pages 12, 13, 28, 29, 41, 55, 67, 76, 86, 96 (all © Lennart Nilsson); by Stephen Oliver on pages 30–31, 32–33, 64–65. **Illustrations** by David Ashby on page 49; by Mark Iley on pages 28, 40, 54, 66–67, 76–77, 86–87, 96–97, 106–107, 120–121; by Tony Randall on pages 12, 34, 35, 51, 52, 64, 70, 98, 99, 100 ("Latching On" line artwork overlay), 110. All other illustrations by Michael Grimsdale.